McGraw-Hill Clinical Care Plans

Perinatal/Neonatal Nursing

Notice

Medicine is an ever-changing science. As new research and clinical experience broaden our knowledge, changes in treatment and drug therapy are required. The authors, editor, and publisher of this work have checked with sources believed to be reliable in their efforts to provide information that is complete and generally in accord with the standards accepted at the time of publication. However, in view of the possibility of human error or changes in medical sciences, neither the editors nor the publisher nor any other party who has been involved in the preparation or publication of this work warrants that the information contained herein is in every respect accurate or complete, and they are not responsible for any errors or omissions or for the results obtained from the use of such information. Readers are encouraged to confirm the information contained herein with other sources. For example and in particular, readers are advised to check the product information sheet included in the package of each drug they plan to administer to be certain that the information contained in this book is accurate and that changes have not been made in the recommended dose or in the contraindications for administration. This recommendation is of particular importance in connection with new or infrequently used drugs.

McGraw-Hill Clinical Care Plans

Perinatal/Neonatal Nursing

Marlene Mayers, RN, MS
Series Editor

Consultant, Nursing Practice / Administration

Annette Jacobson, RN, MSN
Associate Editor

Perinatal Clinical Nurse Specialist

McGraw-Hill, Inc.
Health Professions Division

New York St. Louis San Francisco Auckland Bogotá Caracas Lisbon London Madrid Mexico City Milan Montreal New Delhi San Juan Singapore Sydney Tokyo Toronto

McGraw-Hill Clinical Care Plans: Perinatal/Neonatal Nursing

1234567890 MALMAL 9987654

ISBN: 0-07-105463-4
ISSN: 1074-4231

The editors were Gail Gavert and Mariapaz Ramos Englis; the production supervisor was Gyl Favours; the text design and production was by Beneda Design. Malloy Lithographing was printer and binder.

This book is printed on acid-free paper.

To perinatal and neonatal nurses who care for the health and well-being of infants and families.

CONTENTS

CONTENTS

REVIEWERS AND CONTRIBUTORS

CLINICAL REVIEWERS

Roxanne M. Cole, RN, C, ADN
Staff Nurse
Neonatal

Denice Goodheart, RN, BSN
Staff Nurse
Neonatal

Bren Groves, RN, MN
Nurse Educator
Pediatric Critical Care

Chris Heritage, RN, C, BSN
Staff Nurse
Perinatal

Mary Henrikson, RN, C, MSN
Director of Nursing
Maternal/Child

Susan M. Howson, RN, C, MSN
Nurse
Neonatal Outreach

Patricia Robin McCartney, RN, C, MSN
Clinical Assistant Professor and
Staff Nurse, Labor & Delivery Unit

Julia E. Orosz, RN, C, MSN
Regional Education Coordinator
Perinatal

Sigrid Stephens, RN, C, MSN
NICU Education Coordinator,
Neonatal Development Specialist

Caryn Wood, RN, C, BSN
Staff Nurse
Perinatal

CONTRIBUTORS

Vicky L. Armstrong, RN, C, MSN
CNS, Perinatal Outreach Program
Children's Hospital
Columbus, Ohio

Andrea M. Arnett, RN, CS, MS
Nurse Manager, NICU/Perinatal
Kaiser Permanente Medical Center
Hayward, California

Ellyn H. Bell, RN, CPNP, MA
CNS, OB/GYN Division, Newborn Nursery
University of Iowa Hospitals & Clinics
Iowa City, Iowa

Ann M. Bickford, RN, C, MS
CNS, Maternal Child Health
Spartanburg Regional Medical Center
Spartanburg, South Carolina

Joea E. Bierchen, RN, MSN, EdD
Professor, Nursing
St. Petersburg Junior College
St. Petersburg, Florida

Kathy Brown, RN, BSN
Lecturer and Lab Coordinator
University of Southern Colorado
Pueblo, Colorado

Sandra Godman Brown, RN, DSN
Assistant Professor, Nursing
Medical University of South Carolina
Charleston, South Carolina

Judith A. Carveth, RN, PhD, CNM
Assistant Professor, Nursing
University of North Carolina
Charlotte, North Carolina

Marilyn J. Chapman, RN, C, MSN
Patient Services Sector,
Support Center Leader, QA/CQI
University of Chicago Hospitals
Chicago, Illinois

Roxanne M. Cole, RN, C, ADN
Staff Nurse
Sacred Heart General Hospital
Eugene, Oregon

Geraldine R. Davis, RN, C, BSN
Staff Development Specialist
Parkview Episcopal Medical Center
Pueblo, Colorado

Geraldine Diemer, RN, PhD
Clinical Associate Professor, Nursing
Univeirsity of Wisconsin
Madison, Wisconsin

Nancy Jane Donoho, RN, C, MSN
CNS, Maternal/Infant
Fort Sanders Health System
Knoxville, Tennessee

Margaret Evelyn-Pinkser, RN, C, MA
Instructor, Staff Development
& Continuing Education
Maimonides Medical Center
Brooklyn, New York

Debra Cunningham Facello, RN, C, MSN
Perinatal Specialist
Kent State University
East Liverpool, Ohio

Willa Hill Fuller, RN, C, BSN
Educational Coordinator
Medical/Surgical Services
Orlando Regional Healthcare System
Orlando, Florida

Denice Goodheart, RN, BSN
Staff Nurse
Sacred Heart General Hospital
Eugene, Oregon

Bren Groves, RN, MN
Nurse Educator
Sacred Heart General Hospital
Eugene, Oregon

Julie E. Harrell, RN, C, BSN
Clinical Nurse IV
Children's Hospital
Columbus, Ohio

Chris Heritage, RN, C, BSN
Staff Nurse
Sacred Heart General Hospital
Eugene, Oregon

Mary Henrikson, RN, C, MSN
Director, Maternal/Child Nursing
Salem Hospital
Salem, Orgeon

Michelle R. Hicks, RN, BSN
Clinical Nurse III
C.S. Mott Children's Hospital
University of Michigan Medical Center
Ann Arbor, Michigan

CONTRIBUTORS

Rometta M. Hock, RN, MSN
Instructor, Nursing
University of Alabama
Huntsville, Alabama

Susan M. Howson, RN, C, MSN
Nurse, Neonatal Outreach
Children's Hospital Medical Center of Akron
Akron, Ohio

Linda A. Hunter-Klein, RN, C, BSN
Staff Instructor, LDR
Nursing Research and Development
Women & Infants' Hospital
Providence, Rhode Island

Vicky Janos, RN, MSN
Assistant Professor, Nursing
University of Southern Colorado
Pueblo, Colorado

Nadine A. Kassity, RN, BSN
Educator, Neonatal Outreach
Children's Hospital and Health Center
San Diego, California

Margaret Konefal, RN, Phd
Director, Critical Care Nursing
Children's Hospital
Columbus, Ohio

Mary L. Krywanio, RN, DNS
Director, Nursing Education & Research
St. Louis Children's Hospital
St. Louis, Missouri

Cdr. Mary M. Leemhuis, RN, BS
Assistant Chief Nurse/Nurse Educator
U.S. Public Health Service
Carl Albert Indian Health Facility
Ada, Oklahoma

Carol A. Loan, RN, CPNP, MA
CNS, OB/GYN Division, Newborn Nursery
University of Iowa Hospitals & Clinics
Iowa City, Iowa

Patricia Robin McCartney, RN, C, MSN
Clinical Assistant Professor, Nursing
State University of New York
Staff Nurse, Labor & Delivery
Children's Hospital of Buffalo
Buffalo, New York

Debra Vidrine McCauley, RN, MSN
Instructor, Nursing
Louisiana State University
Eunice, Louisiana

Theresa A. Marvelli, RN, C, BSN, MA
Instructor
Maimonides Medical Center
Brooklyn, New York

Julia E. Orosz, RN, C, MSN
Education Coordinator
Regional Perinatal
Children's Hospital Medical Center of Akron
Akron, Ohio

Janet L. Owens, RN, C, MSN
Nursing Outreach Coordinator
Nursing Education & Research
St. Louis Children's Hospital
St. Louis, Missouri

Kathleen Palange, RN, C, MS
Assistant Director, Nursing
L.S. Packard Children's Hospital at Stanford
Palo Alto, California

Carol J. Pankratz, RN, MSN
CNS, Medical-Surgical
Sacred Heart General Hospital
Eugene, Oregon

Carol L. Pattillo, RN, C, BSN
Nurse Educator, Perinatal
University of California
Irvine Medical Center
Orange, California

Joanette Pete-McGadney, RN, PhD
Assistant Dean and Associate Professor
Texas Woman's University
Dallas, Texas

Duayna Pucci, RN, CNA, MSN
Assistant Director, Hospital Nursing
Kaiser Medical Center
Hayward, California

Sandra Raymer-Raff, MS, RN, C
Lecturer and CNS, Perinatal
San Jose State University
San Jose, California

Christine Sadinski, RN, CS, MSN
Senior Nursing Instructor
Children's Hospital Medical Center of Akron
Akron, Ohio

Monica E. Steele, RN, C, MS, BS
CNS, Perinatal
Maimonides Medical Center
Brooklyn, New York

Sigrid Stephens, RN, C, MSN
Education Coordinator, NICU
Specialist, Neonatal Development
Children's Hospital Medical Center of Akron
Akron, Ohio

Stephanie Stewart, RN, MSN, PhD
Associate Professor
University of Wisconsin
Oshkosh, Wisconsin

Nadiji Struble, RN, BA
Chief Nurse Executive
Women's Hospital
Las Vegas, Nevada

Ermilina S. Villegas, RN, C, BSN
Nurse Clinician
Medical Center Hospital
Odessa, Texas

Caryn Wood, RN, C, BSN
Staff Nurse
Sacred Heart General Hospital
Eugene, Oregon

PREFACE

THE McGRAW-HILL CLINICAL CARE PLAN SERIES

This book and its companions in the McGraw-Hill Clinical Care Plan series are the most current editions of the now "classic" Standard Nursing Care Plans that were first published by Mayers/El Camino in the mid-seventies. These books, in frequently updated versions, have been published continuously since that time. In those early years, as the first of their kind, they did much to stimulate nursing's early development of formalized, systematic care planning/evaluation systems in hospitals throughout most English-speaking countries. Today they continue to be a part of nursing's continuing effort to articulate and advance the knowledge base of nursing. In addition, metric conversions have been given as appropriate to facilitate global audiences.

These new editions, now published by McGraw-Hill, preserve all of the most preferred features of previous editions. They also contain many enhancements in format and style which make them even easier to use than ever before. The content has benefited from the contributions of a greater number, and wider range, of nurse caregivers, specialists, and educators than there were before.

These books maintain continuity with previous editions through oversight by the same Series Editor, Marlene Mayers. In addition, a new Associate Editor, Annette Jacobson, has been added to the editorial team for this book, *Perinatal/Neonatal Nursing*. She is a clinical nurse specialist and clinical educator for the maternal-child department of a large regional medical center.

This editorial team, in close collaboration with panels of clinical reviewers, have combined their talents to produce these definitive books of nursing care plans for the acute care setting.

The books in the McGraw-Hill Clinical Care Plan series are: *Perinatal/Neonatal Nursing, Pediatric Nursing, Medical-Surgical Nursing*. They are specifically designed to be used by nurses in the hospital setting. The three books address the acute problems that are experienced by many people at some time during their lives: before birth, through childhood, and into adulthood. These problems frequently result in hospitalization where nurses, as the predominant caregivers, provide the moment-by-moment care that assesses, nurtures, and guides them through their acute crises.

Guides for Care Planning in the Hospital Setting

These books are entitled "Clinical Care Plans" because they are carefully written in the succinct style associated with the clinical setting. They help nurses and students visualize how a functional care plan might be phrased. Some of these plans contain more items of information than a nurse might normally need for a specific patient, but they offer groups or combinations of activities from which to select the most relevant items. By referring to these already carefully crafted documents, and by adding the necessary qualifying words and phrases, a nurse can thereby efficiently produce care plans that contain both standardized and carefully individualized elements.

The plans' format is the familiar three-column design. Terminology is consistent with what is actually written in charts and on care plans in the clinical setting. Terms are succinct enough so that, with only minor modification, they can be entered into a critical pathway, a flow sheet, or into computerized information systems.

Each book includes the most commonly occurring medical diagnoses (or topics of concern) that are experienced by patients admitted to that clinical area.

Familiar Phraseology

Phraseology tends to conform to generally familiar hospital nursing form and style practices. (1) Nursing Diagnoses are those developed by NANDA; (2) Outcome Criteria include action verbs that direct attention to those measurable/observable phenomena (subjective and objective) that make evaluation possible;
(3) Interventions (groups/combinations of nursing activities) are phrased as directives.

Because these plans are meant to be used in the acute care setting, their terms are those of hospital nurses. Brief and succinct phrases are used rather than sentences. Outcome criteria are written in the present tense, active voice. Symbols and abbreviations common to the hospital setting are used.

Easy to Individualize

These care plans are easy to individualize because they are carefully crafted to apply to specific clinical situations. For example, the management of "Fluid Volume Deficit" (a NANDA diagnosis) for a child with leukemia will differ from fluid volume management for an adult or child with an eating disorder. Or, for example, "Altered Nutrition: Less than body requirements" is treated differently in the care plan for diabetes mellitus than it is in that for a child with biliary atresia or for an infant with cleft palate.

It is also within the individualization process that the patient's collaboration becomes vital. Involvement empowers people to become competent and knowledgeable about their health, and, thus, to become effective on their own behalf. Including the patient and family in reviewing, understanding, and amending the plan of care can make a significant difference in the outcomes of that care. It can also influence patients' long-term healthcare practices.

Excellent Reference Tools

The books are designed to be used on a daily basis. They provide easy to find information about clinical nursing care. When kept near at hand, for instance on the nursing unit as well as in school and hospital libraries, they serve as reminder systems – as do other reference texts and manuals. They are excellent references to use when nurses are reviewing literature as part of the periodic updates of their own standard nursing care plans.

A Clinical Care Plan prompts a nurse to address all of the relevant issues for a patient's care. It is difficult, when under the pressures of an acute care setting, to rely on human memory to recall each and every one of the variables to be addressed in a patient's situation. A responsible professional in any field uses "lists and prompts" to bolster human memory. Every caregiver, too, needs various kinds of reference and reminder systems to provide safe and effective care. Clinical Care Plans are among the best of them.

Excellent Learning Tools

The clearly organized format and graphic nonlinear design make these books excellent learning tools for hospital or school instruction. Each care plan illuminates the logic that underlies nursing practice. Nursing Diagnoses and etiologies along with their outcome criteria are specified. These, in turn, trigger groups or combinations of nursing activities that are understood to prevent, ameliorate, or resolve the underlying problems. The graphic format structures and organizes these units of information. Their relationships are made clear.

This logical framework helps students to more easily understand and to integrate the detailed information found in their major nursing texts.

Outcome Criteria for Quality Assurance/Improvement

Included are many outcome criteria that are directly linked to care assessment for quality enhancement. Clinical Care Plans typically offer several outcome criteria for each nursing diagnosis. Criteria are phrased in specific, measurable terms.

These care plans express commonly understood outcome and process criteria and thereby provide an excellent device for measuring quality and identifying accountability. With only minor modification they can be utilized as the source of outcome and process criteria for patient care evaluation tools such as those used in Total Quality Management (TQM), chart reviews, concurrent reviews, patient surveys, and so on.

Practice-Based Development

These books are the result of a process of collaboration among nurse clinicians, caregivers, and educators from across the country. Through this process, standards and practices have become integrated into a carefully organized, inductively developed, practice-based whole. Yet, each book also clearly reflects the differing nursing cultures and voices that are unique to each clinical area.

Our goal has been to provide care plans that specifically address the needs of hospitalized patients. And we respectfully acknowledge the extraordinary commitment and skill of their caregivers: today's hospital nurses.

Acknowledgments

We wish to thank the following individuals for their extraordinary contributions to manuscript development: Keith Albin, Christine Beneda, Cheryl Hunt, Barbara Land, Penny Allmett, Carol Roth, Peggy Pickens, Sigrid Stephens, Patricia McCartney, Denice Goodheart, Mary Henrikson, Sandi Lederman, Nancy Hoyt, and Bren Groves. A special note of appreciation goes to Shasta Hatter, our manuscript coordinator.

Marlene Mayers, RN, MS
Series Editor

Annette Jacobson, RN, MSN
Associate Editor

McGraw-Hill Clinical Care Plans

Perinatal/Neonatal Nursing

CONTENTS

INSTRUCTIONS

HOW TO USE McGRAW-HILL CLINICAL CARE PLANS

This definitive, easy-to-use reference book provides the hospital nurse or nursing student, with a fast-track approach to patient care planning. The design is easy to read, well-indexed, and gives the reader a jump start in developing an individualized plan of care.

THE FORMAT

The care plans are divided into six categories: Nursing Diagnoses, Outcome Criteria, Interventions, Rationale, Other Less Common Nursing Diagnoses, and Essential Discharge Criteria. Take each category and review the specific components contained within.

Nursing Diagnoses

NANDA nursing diagnoses are used as the standard nomenclature for these care plans. They are listed in the first, or left-hand, column of the care plan as noted below.

EDUCATION FOR DISCHARGE

NURSING DIAGNOSIS	OUTCOME CRITERIA	INTERVENTIONS
1 **Knowledge Deficit (relevant healthcare needs)** *r.t. lack of recall, cognitive limitation, impaired communication, depression, illiteracy, lack of exposure, withdrawal*	• Verbalizes understanding of instructions	• Describe how to use new skills, behaviors in daily living • Use open-ended questions to derive information regarding learning • Simplify information to meet the patient's/family's level of understanding or developmental age

Our example is "Knowledge Deficit" as it appears in our *Education for Discharge* care plan.

Because of shortened lengths of stay in the hospital, all relevant nursing diagnoses likely will be addressed upon admission. Otherwise, the diagnoses may be prioritized according to patient need and nurse judgment. The diagnostic *hunch* can be confirmed by reviewing those diagnoses listed under the topic, since they are most likely to characterize patient problems associated with that particular topic or medical diagnosis. Sometimes, the reader is referred to other care plans in the book that may help develop a particular plan or address a specific issue, such as *pain* or *education for discharge*.

The last part of the diagnostic statement is the etiology, or list of risk factors, that follows the "related to" phrase as shown. We have chosen to abbreviate the "related to" statement to ***r.t.*** within each care plan. A variety of potential etiology statements are listed to get you going. You will want to select the specific etiology for your patient as you begin to develop an individualized plan of care.

For example, Knowledge Deficit might be related to "lack of recall" for one patient, to "cognitive limitation" for another, to "illiteracy" for a third patient.

Clearly, the different etiologies would require different teaching-learning interventions.

EDUCATION FOR DISCHARGE

NURSING DIAGNOSIS	OUTCOME CRITERIA	INTERVENTIONS
1 **Knowledge Deficit (relevant healthcare needs)** *r.t. lack of recall, cognitive limitation, impaired communication, depression, illiteracy, lack of exposure, withdrawal*	• Verbalizes understanding of instructions	• Describe how to use new skills, behaviors in daily living • Use open-ended questions to derive information regarding learning • Simplify information to meet the patient's/family's level of understanding or developmental age

Outcome Criteria

The next column addresses *Outcome Criteria* which is the term chosen to reflect the goals for the patient. Here you will find the patient outcomes anticipated for the certain nursing diagnoses. The outcome, which is written in specific terms, may address the patient and/or family.

These objective and subjective criteria are written in terms of measurable patient behaviors, and each criterion identifies the patient's goals by the time of discharge. Similarly, outcome criteria include objective and subjective parameters that describe successful resolution of the nursing diagnoses.

Because the length of stay in today's acute care setting is compressed, all outcome criteria should be met during the patient's hospital stay. For clarity and simplicity, outcomes have not been separated into short- or long-term phrases. However, care plans can be used as guides for critical pathways or care maps by assigning daily goals, determined by institutional preferences and regional population needs.

You will find that the term *within normal limits* (WNL) has been used to allow for the variation of normal. That variation may be normal for that patient, i.e., return to baseline, or preadmission status. Or normal may reflect the variation within the literature. And it can reflect the variation between institutions or physician preferences for monitoring response to treatment.

EDUCATION FOR DISCHARGE

NURSING DIAGNOSIS	OUTCOME CRITERIA	INTERVENTIONS
1 Knowledge Deficit (relevant healthcare needs) *r.t. lack of recall, cognitive limitation, impaired communication, depression, illiteracy, lack of exposure, withdrawal*	• Verbalizes understanding of instructions	• Describe how to use new [illegible] behaviors in daily living • Use open-ended questions to derive information regarding learning • Simplify information to meet the patient's/family's level of understanding or developmental age

Interventions

Nursing actions are listed in the third column. *Interventions* identify independent and interdependent strategies designed to facilitate or accomplish the outcome criteria. Interventions are specific enough to ensure that established standards of clinical practice are met, yet general enough to allow for institutional preferences. Monitoring and assessment strategies are listed to guide the nurse in ascertaining that outcomes have been met.

Actions listed are both independent and interdependent. Suggestions for referrals are stated when the plan of care may require the expertise of another healthcare discipline. The care plan format can be easily adapted to document which interventions were provided by each discipline. For instance, the nurse can reinforce the plans set forth by the social worker, while saving time in redundant efforts.

In this column you may find the term *within parameters*. This term was chosen to address those assessments that a physician or other primary care provider may state as an acceptable range of normal, such as in blood gases or blood glucose levels. (You may want to refer to the appendixes for normative data.)

Many plans include specific teaching content to correct knowledge deficits and enhance important self-care strategies. You may want to refer to the *Education for Discharge* care plan to supplement this section.

Rationale

Listed at the end of the *Intervention* column you will find *Rationale* for the interventions as they relate to the nursing diagnosis and etiologies. These statements are simple, concise, and offer key concepts to use in researching these concepts further.

EDUCATION FOR DISCHARGE

NURSING DIAGNOSIS	OUTCOME CRITERIA	INTERVENTIONS
	• Participates in care activities	• Establish an environment that enables patient/family to gain control • Build on patient's developmental and learning level; consult with expert as indicated
		RATIONALE: *Learning activities that are geared to the patient's/family's level of prior experience, knowledge, and developmental level are likely to produce positive cognitive behavior changes that are relevant to healthcare needs. Repetition, participation, and graphic/written cues and lists foster learning and recall.*

Other Less Common Nursing Diagnoses

Next you will find that we have included a listing of other diagnoses that tend to be associated with the medical diagnosis or problem. These diagnoses may also reflect other potential problems that patients with this medical condition present in the acute care setting.

You will see that etiologies have been omitted from the diagnostic statement, allowing for individual variations in patient assessment by the nurse. These additional nursing diagnoses, supported by a particular patient's characteristics and etiology, can be developed through the nursing process.

We refer to these diagnoses as "less common" because they are less likely to be addressed during a brief hospital stay. However, these nursing diagnoses may be commonly addressed with complications or in the outpatient or home care setting.

Essential Discharge Criteria

The final section in each care plan is the *Essential Discharge Criteria*. Here you will find that we have broadly summarized the Outcome Criteria contained within the care plan. The outcome criteria have been collapsed into essential aspects that

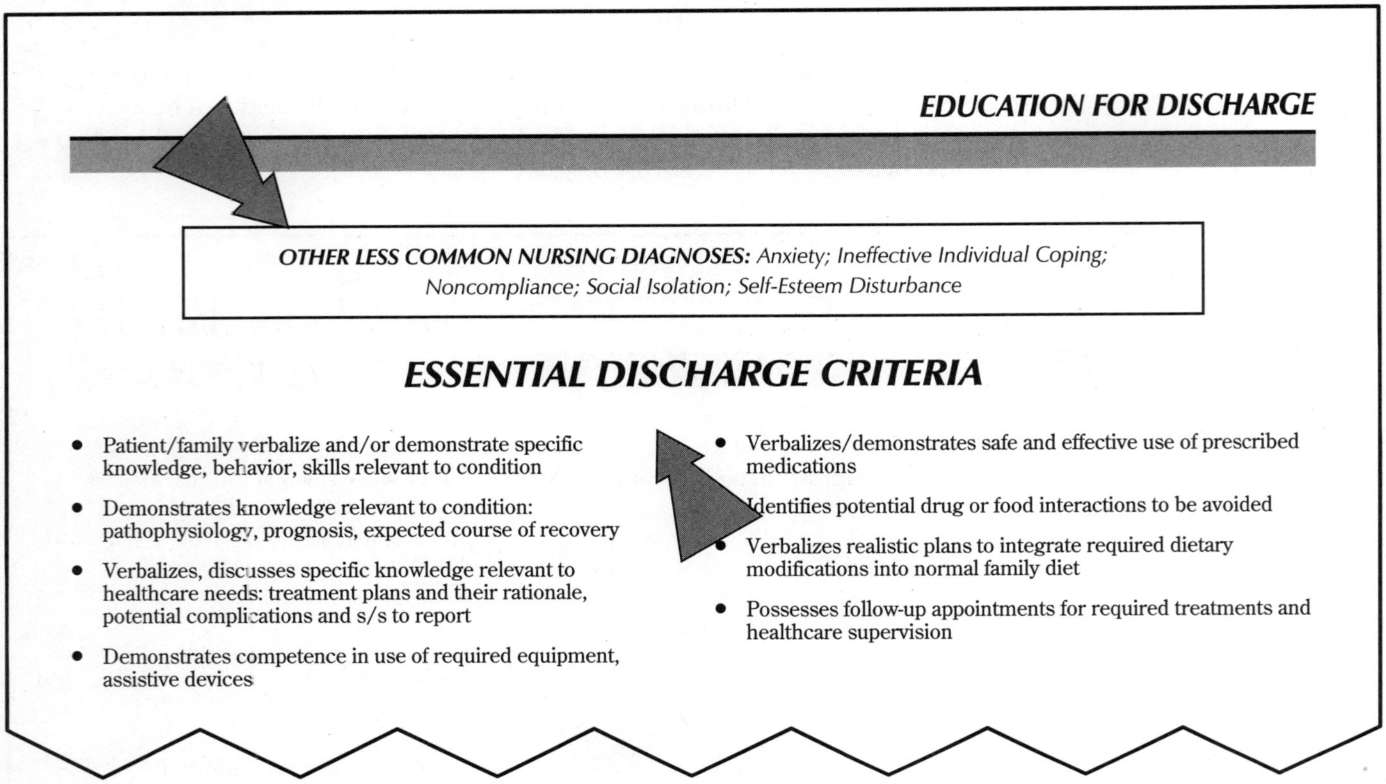

EDUCATION FOR DISCHARGE

OTHER LESS COMMON NURSING DIAGNOSES: *Anxiety; Ineffective Individual Coping; Noncompliance; Social Isolation; Self-Esteem Disturbance*

ESSENTIAL DISCHARGE CRITERIA

- Patient/family verbalize and/or demonstrate specific knowledge, behavior, skills relevant to condition
- Demonstrates knowledge relevant to condition: pathophysiology, prognosis, expected course of recovery
- Verbalizes, discusses specific knowledge relevant to healthcare needs: treatment plans and their rationale, potential complications and s/s to report
- Demonstrates competence in use of required equipment, assistive devices
- Verbalizes/demonstrates safe and effective use of prescribed medications
- Identifies potential drug or food interactions to be avoided
- Verbalizes realistic plans to integrate required dietary modifications into normal family diet
- Possesses follow-up appointments for required treatments and healthcare supervision

must be present to allow for a safe and effective discharge from the acute care setting.

For example, you will notice that we have assumed that basic physiologic function is present but we will speak to the need for "resolution of respiratory compromise" for the patient who was admitted with pneumonia. You won't necessarily find discussion of HR WNL, BP WNL, or bowel function WNL, since these are only indirectly related to the presenting problem. And maybe that patient has a superimposed cardiac abnormality that will not be ameliorated by the care provided during the bout with pneumonia.

Additionally, we incorporated JCAHO requirements regarding discharge. You will find strategies to ensure compliance in the *Education for Discharge* plan, which addresses Knowledge Deficit.

GETTING STARTED

Now that you have an understanding of the layout and content, it's time to get started developing your individualized care plan.

- Select the medical diagnoses you are interested in and turn to the standard care plan.
- Identify the nursing diagnosis relevant to your patient based on your assessment. Remember to review the *Other Less Common Nursing Diagnoses* section for other potential diagnoses.

- Select the appropriate etiology for each nursing diagnosis.
- Identify outcome criteria specific to the etiology demonstrated by the patient.
- Review the essential discharge criteria to ensure inclusion of essential aspects.
- List interventions necessary to facilitate achieving the identified outcomes as they relate to the patient.
- Review the plan of care with the patient and family and revise as needed.
- Implement the plan of care, communicating with other healthcare providers.
- Evaluate the patient's progress toward attaining the outcome criteria; revise the plan as needed.
- Identify variances for developing Improvement of Organizational Program (quality assurance).

HELPFUL HINTS

A successful plan begins with a solid nursing admission data base. Objective and subjective information is clustered to determine whether or not defining characteristics support a particular nursing diagnosis.

You will not find *exact* wording from care plan to care plan concerning a specific nursing diagnoses, e.g., impaired skin integrity. This is intentional, providing the reader with a variety of phrasing options. (It's also less boring that way!)

You will find the term *family* is used broadly to describe persons significant to the patient. These persons may be mother, brother, father, aunt, neighbor, friend, or any other "significant other."

For diagnoses that tend to span age groups, such as meningitis, the reader needs to incorporate developmental considerations as indicated. Additionally, the diagnosis may occur across the life span, and these developmental "passages" should be considered as well.

Achievement of Essential Discharge Criteria should be addressed and documented as part of the discharge notation. The behaviors listed are those that the patient must demonstrate before safely leaving the hospital. The nurse obtains data from ongoing patient assessment, return demonstrations, and the patient record to evaluate whether outcome criteria have been met. If the criteria are not met, appropriate referrals should be made and documented to ensure care continuity after discharge.

Appendixes may be helpful to you when looking for abbreviations, normal lab values, listing of NANDA nursing diagnoses, definitions of medical problems, or defining characteristics of NANDA diagnoses.

EDUCATION FOR DISCHARGE

NURSING DIAGNOSES	OUTCOME CRITERIA	INTERVENTIONS
1 Knowledge Deficit (relevant healthcare needs) *r.t. lack of recall, cognitive limitation, impaired communication, illiteracy, lack of exposure, withdrawal, depression*	• Verbalizes understanding of instructions	• Describe how to use new skills, behaviors in daily living • Use open-ended questions to derive information regarding learning • Simplify information to meet the patient's/family's level of understanding or developmental age
	• Demonstrates appropriate decision-making	• Discuss healthcare needs and methods to achieve success • Teach use of cues to remember health actions • Assess knowledge deficit at every interaction • Consult as needed to develop appropriate teaching plan for patient/family with neurologic learning deficits
	• Assumes responsibility for own learning	• Contact patient/family to provide support; evaluate learning
	• Participates in care activities	• Establish an environment that enables patient/family to gain control • Build on patient's developmental and learning level; consult with expert as indicated
	• Possesses phone numbers for emergency medical help	• Provide opportunities for patient/family to be actively involved in learning • Assess satisfaction with education plan • Provide written materials to reinforce teaching

RATIONALE: *Learning activities that are geared to the patient's/family's level of prior experience, knowledge, and developmental level are likely to produce positive cognitive behavior changes that are relevant to healthcare needs. Repetition, participation, and graphic/written cues and lists foster learning and recall.*

NURSING DIAGNOSES	OUTCOME CRITERIA	INTERVENTIONS
2 Knowledge Deficit (specific knowledge, skills, behaviors) *r.t. lack of future orientation, impaired communication, anger, insufficient maturation to comprehend, refusal to listen*	• Demonstrates skills, behaviors correctly	• Provide information at level of learner's understanding • Utilize self-care protocols and/or instructional packets (as available)
	• Demonstrates ability to perform care	• Set clear learning goals • Utilize motivational techniques to assist patient/family to self-identify necessity of skill
	• Asks questions; seeks clarification	• Provide opportunity to review process or concepts related to skills, behaviors • Discuss realistic expectations to assist in guiding learning
	• Makes realistic statements about expected course, recovery, prognosis	• Offer peer support network or opportunity to observe others successfully mastering care skills and symptom control • Facilitate sense of mastery of skills, behaviors, attitudes
		RATIONALE: *Mutual goal-setting, positive feedback, and return demonstrations motivate the learner to gain desired competencies. The support of significant others also fosters motivation.*
3 Knowledge Deficit (medications) *r.t. lack of exposure, irrational beliefs, need to make sense of life-threatening disease, inability to recall*	• Acquires knowledge of medication administration - lists medications - discusses dosages, effects, side effects	• Provide opportunity to gain sense of control - provide instruction in several modalities • Anticipate and provide assists when sensory or psychomotor limitations are present
	• Verbalizes knowledge of complications	• Provide written and/or audiovisual materials to enable review by patient/family as needed
	• Lists reportable s/s	• Assess patient's/family's acceptance of diagnosis • If available, help patient/family to learn computerized monitoring systems, e.g., OneTouch, Accucheck

NURSING DIAGNOSES	OUTCOME CRITERIA	INTERVENTIONS
		• Discuss sign of decrease in symptoms and/or improvement in health state
	• Discusses rationale for treatment	• Use patient's/family's ideas about illness as a starting point for education and/or training
		RATIONALE: *Use of various teaching-learning modalities that stimulate cognitive, affective, and motor abilities reinforces new and accurate information. Clear, specific information, accompanied by cues and lists, fosters recall of important information.*
4 Knowledge Deficit (diet) *r.t. lack of interest in learning, lack of belief in efficacy of treatment, decreased motivation to learn, misinterpretation of information*	• Demonstrates prescribed diet planning - selects indicated foods from list - recognizes contraindicated foods	• Describe problem-solving process to assist patient/family to integrate diet plan • Discuss with other healthcare providers the need to actively involve patient/family in decision-making • Establish an environment conducive to learning - free of distraction - with visual aids and diet lists • Teach how to provide rewards for maintenance of positive health behaviors
	• Verbalizes knowledge of follow-up appointments	• Reinforce utilization of information gained - include support persons in integration of information • Teach patient/family how to find, use, and evaluate community resources - education - support - treatment

NURSING DIAGNOSES	OUTCOME CRITERIA	INTERVENTIONS
	• Copes adequately	• Discuss plans for patient/family to include health behaviors identified as valuable to self • Set clear, mutually agreed-upon learning goals • Be accessible to patient/family to reinforce teaching
		RATIONALE: *Involvement in anticipatory problem-solving and planning raises likelihood of effective problem-solving after discharge. Discussion by patient and family of coping strengths and healthcare goals raises the likelihood of a continuation of this kind of support network. Discussion and support foster effective behavior changes.*
5 Knowledge Deficit (equipment) *r.t. excessive anxiety, need to follow new and/or complex treatment, unfamiliarity with information*	• Demonstrates competence in equipment use	• Teach how to mentally and physically rehearse skill • Describe how mastery meets patient's/family's own standard for adequate coping
	• Possesses phone numbers for equipment and supplies	• Demonstrate to patient/family how to use equipment and obtain services • Discuss where to access supplies and/or equipment; provide written information
	• Demonstrates required skills related to supplies required	• Assist with practice of skill until performance shows mastery and confidence
	• Verbalizes understanding of instructions	• Check with patient/family often during teaching to elicit and evaluate understanding
		RATIONALE: *Demonstration and return demonstration with positive, supportive feedback enhance motor skill mastery.*

OTHER LESS COMMON NURSING DIAGNOSES: *Anxiety; Ineffective Individual Coping; Noncompliance; Social Isolation; Self-Esteem Disturbance*

ESSENTIAL DISCHARGE CRITERIA

- Patient/family verbalize and/or demonstrate specific knowledge, behavior, skills relevant to condition
- Demonstrates knowledge relevant to condition: pathophysiology, prognosis, expected course of recovery
- Verbalizes, discusses specific knowledge relevant to healthcare needs: treatment plans and their rationale; potential complications and s/s to report
- Demonstrates competence in use of required equipment, assistive devices
- Verbalizes/demonstrates safe and effective use of prescribed medications
- Identifies potential drug or food interactions to be avoided
- Verbalizes realistic plans to integrate required dietary modifications into normal family diet
- Possesses follow-up appointments for required treatments and healthcare supervision

ANTEPARTUM

CONTENTS

ABRUPTIO PLACENTAE

NURSING DIAGNOSES	OUTCOME CRITERIA	INTERVENTIONS
1 Pain *r.t. irritation of uterine muscle by retroplacental bleeding, uterine contractions*	• Displays increased comfort - relaxation of face and extremities	• Assess location and character of pain • Assess contraction pattern, resting tone, and localized tenderness
	• Verbalizes increased comfort	• Position for comfort (but not supine) • Provide or assist with analgesic/anesthetic as prescribed • Provide comfort measures, support with pillows • Instruct/implement relaxation techniques • Reduce/modify environmental stimuli
		RATIONALE: *Monitor to detect improvement/worsening of pain and response to therapeutic plan. Reduce physical, emotional, and environmental stimuli that contribute to pain.*
2 Altered Tissue Perfusion (maternal) *r.t. blood loss*	• Displays adequate tissue perfusion - improved/stable VS - skin warm	• Assess for signs of shock: VS; I&O; skin for color and warmth; CRT qh or more often as indicated • Assess amount of blood loss (measure blood on perineal pads and underpads) • Assess contraction pattern and resting tone • Assess uterine activity and abdominal tenderness • Measure and mark fundal height on the abdomen • Review diagnostic studies (H&H, clotting studies) • Observe for signs of DIC
	• Shows no s/s of hypoxia - no pallor or cyanosis - CRT < 3 sec - BP WNL	• Provide O_2 by face mask as prescribed • Maintain patient on bed rest • Avoid supine hypotension by keeping mother on side or wedged to the left

NURSING DIAGNOSES	OUTCOME CRITERIA	INTERVENTIONS
		• Prepare for emergency C/S if indicated
		RATIONALE: *Monitor improvement/worsening of tissue perfusion and response to therapeutic plan. Adequate tissue perfusion is dependent on oxygenated blood reaching the cells.*
3 Impaired Gas Exchange (fetal) *r.t. disruption of placental attachment, impaired blood flow to fetus* *(Refer to "Fetal Stress" care plan)*	• Exhibits adequate fetal oxygenation - normal FHR baseline (120-160 bpm) - absence of late decelerations - presence of good FHR variability	• Assess fetal response through continuous electronic fetal monitoring • Administer O_2 to mother by face mask as prescribed • Avoid supine hypotension and poor placental perfusion by keeping mother on side or wedged to the left • Prepare for neonatal resuscitation utilizing Neonatal Resuscitation Program guidelines
	• Exhibits normal fetal activity	• Assess fetal activity • Estimate gestational age
	• Shows no evidence of meconium in amniotic fluid	• Assess color of amniotic fluid (port wine; meconium staining) • Assist with fetal capillary blood samples
		RATIONALE: *Monitor improvement/worsening of fetal oxygenation status and response to therapeutic plan. Increase O^2 saturation of the blood.*

ANTEPARTUM

NURSING DIAGNOSES	OUTCOME CRITERIA	INTERVENTIONS
4 Fluid Volume Deficit *r.t. bleeding between placenta and uterine wall*	• Exhibits adequate circulating volume - output not < 30 mL/h - VS WNL	• Assess VS, I&O qh or more often as indicated • Assess urinary sp. gr. q2-4h
	• Displays adequate hydration - skin moist with good turgor - mucous membranes moist	• Assess skin turgor and mucous membranes
	• Maintains Hb, Hct WNL	• Review data from diagnostic studies (H&H) • Assess blood loss (uterine: covert or overt bleeding) • Administer fluid and blood replacement as prescribed
		RATIONALE: *Monitor fluid status and response to therapeutic plan to prevent adverse effects of hypovolemia.*
5 Anxiety *r.t. uncertain maternal and fetal prognosis*	• Displays reduced anxiety - verbalizes fewer anxieties - relaxed face and extremities - uses adaptive coping measures	• Assess coping styles and support systems of client and family • Have client identify concerns and fears • Keep client and family informed of maternal and fetal status and therapeutic plan • Reinforce positive aspects of health • Encourage questions and open communication • Promote client decision-making whenever possible • Encourage verbalization of fears and concerns
		RATIONALE: *These measures help recognize current level of anxiety and resources available for coping. Information fosters problem-solving.*

NURSING DIAGNOSES	OUTCOME CRITERIA	INTERVENTIONS
6 Knowledge Deficit *r.t. initial experience with abruptio placentae*	• Verbalizes adequate knowledge base - accurate understanding of clinical situation and therapeutic plan	• Provide factual information regarding current status and therapeutic plan • Allow opportunity for questions by patient and family
		RATIONALE: *Accurate information promotes sound decision-making and trust in care providers.*

OTHER LESS COMMON NURSING DIAGNOSES: *Anticipatory Grieving; High Risk for Injury; High Risk for Infection; Altered Sexuality Patterns; Caregiver Role Strain; Impaired Home Maintenance Management*

ESSENTIAL DISCHARGE CRITERIA

- Maintains stable normal VS
- Displays no pallor or cyanosis
- Shows Hb, Hct, clotting studies WNL
- Demonstrates FHR WNL
- Verbalizes plans for follow-up care, lists reportable s/s

CANCER

NURSING DIAGNOSES	OUTCOME CRITERIA	INTERVENTIONS
1 Anxiety *r.t. diagnosis of cancer, uncertain future expectations*	• Displays reduced anxiety - verbalizes anxieties	• Encourage patient to identify concerns and fears • Assess patient's coping ability, support systems, and understanding of condition and therapeutic plan
	• Uses adaptive coping measures	• Provide time to be with patient • Encourage family and friends to maintain frequent contact through visiting patient, telephone calls, letters/cards • Instruct patient regarding relaxation techniques • Assist patient to develop care goals and make decisions regarding care
		RATIONALE: *These measures help client recognize current level of anxiety and resources available for coping. Making decisions promotes sense of control and reduces anxieties.*
2 Anticipatory Grieving *r.t. perceived loss of body structure, functional ability, and/or fetus*	• Accepts body changes or functional abilities - verbalizes and accepts the perceived loss	• Discuss the concept of loss and the grieving process with patient and family • Assist patient to identify and verbalize the anticipated loss and how it will affect her life • Assess patient coping ability and support systems
	• Shares grief with family and significant others	• Provide time for listening to patient's concerns • Acknowledge the depth of the grief • Encourage family or significant others to support client • Provide privacy for grieving • Refer patient/family to secular and spiritual support groups
		RATIONALE: *Loss must be acknowledged before grieving can begin. People progress through the grief process at different rates.*

NURSING DIAGNOSES	OUTCOME CRITERIA	INTERVENTIONS
3 Body Image Disturbance *r.t. loss of body structure or function with surgery, chemotherapy, or radiation therapy*	• Accepts changed body image - expresses positive feelings regarding self	• Accept client's self-perception of the loss • Assess coping abilities • Encourage client to voice concerns regarding body/functional ability
	• Participates in care for body area/function altered by cancer and its treatment	• Assist/encourage patient to perform daily activities • Identify stable/improved body functions • Refer to support groups • Assist with hygiene and grooming • Discuss onset of hair loss and time of regrowth if chemotherapeutic agent causes hair loss
		RATIONALE: *A complete data base regarding client self-perceptions and coping ability promotes proper selection of therapeutic interventions and fosters sense of independence and positive feelings regarding self.*
4 Knowledge Deficit *r.t. lack of experience with neoplastic conditions/therapies*	• Verbalizes accurate understanding of clinical situation and therapeutic plan	• Assess patient's knowledge regarding diagnosis, prognosis, and plan of care • Explore with patient and family the meaning and impact of the health alteration on their lives • Provide factual information regarding current status and therapeutic plan • Allow opportunity for questions by client and family
		RATIONALE: *A complete data base regarding client knowledge of health problem and therapies promotes selection of appropriate nursing interventions. An accurate knowledge base promotes sound decision-making and coping for client and family.*

ANTEPARTUM

NURSING DIAGNOSES	OUTCOME CRITERIA	INTERVENTIONS
5 Altered Nutrition: Less than body requirements *r.t. inability to ingest and absorb nutrients*	• Maintains adequate nutritional status - minimizes weight loss or maintains weight	• Assess client's weight weekly • Assess fluid and food preferences and intake • Assess output (urinary, vomitus, stool) • Help client establish goal for desired weight and intake
	• Ingests, retains adequate essential nutrients	• Promote nutritional intake - offer choice in foods whenever possible - maintain pleasant environment for mealtime - maintain good oral hygiene
		RATIONALE: *Provide data base to monitor improvement/worsening of nutritional status and to select appropriate interventions. Preferred foods offered in pleasant surroundings promote ingestion and digestion.*
6 High Risk for Infection *r.t. reduced immunity from chemotherapy or radiation*	• Is free from infection - temperature and pulse WNL - WBC count WNL - wounds/incisions remain clean and continue to heal - absence of diarrhea or skin breakdown	• Instruct patient/family in importance of hygiene, skin care, and avoidance of individuals with infections; s/s of infection • Encourage adequate fluid and nutritional intake • Maintain strict aseptic technique in care of wounds or invasive therapies • Instruct to report any s/s of infection immediately
		RATIONALE: *Preventative measures reduce risk factors for poor healing and invasion of body by pathogens. Early detection and treatment lead to reduced morbidity.*

OTHER LESS COMMON NURSING DIAGNOSIS: *Altered Family Processes; Ineffective Family Coping; Self-Esteem Disturbance; Spiritual Distress; Altered Sexuality Patterns; Impaired Home Maintenance Management*

ESSENTIAL DISCHARGE CRITERIA

- Maintains stability in ingestion and digestion of nutrients
- Has stable support systems for coping with altered body structure and/or functional ability
- Demonstrates FHR WNL for gestation
- Verbalizes accurate understanding of prescribed therapies and has realistic plans to implement them with assistance available in the home

CARDIAC DISEASE

NURSING DIAGNOSES	OUTCOME CRITERIA	INTERVENTIONS
1 Fluid Volume Excess *r.t. pulmonary congestion, renal insufficiency*	• Shows VS, BP WNL for stage of pregnancy	• Assess VS, BP q2-4h as indicated • Assess RR, effort q2-4h and prn • Administer BP medication, chronotropic, alpha pressor agents
	• Exhibits no SOB, dyspnea • Has no edema • Shows CRT < 3 sec	• Monitor for s/s of CHF - SOB - dyspnea - edema - tachycardia - rales - oliguria - decreased O_2 sat - anxiety, restlessness
	• Shows balanced I&O	• Maintain strict I&O • Assess daily weights
	• Na (serum) WNL	• Explain fluid and Na restrictions • Monitor electrolytes
	• Shows normal PT, PTT	• Monitor CBC values, PT, PTT
		RATIONALE: *Identify the early development of pulmonary congestion, which can progress to CHF due to increased preload.*
2 Activity Intolerance *r.t. chronic disease, advanced pregnancy*	• Demonstrates ADL with minimum exertion	• Assess activity tolerance levels • Teach strategies for achieving ADL; demonstrate prescribed limited exercise techniques • Explain rationale for bed rest
	• Shows RR, BP WNL	• Assess RR, BP q2-4h as indicated
		RATIONALE: *Maternal chronic cardiac disease potentiates the effects of advancing pregnancy on physiologic status and energy reserve.*

NURSING DIAGNOSES	OUTCOME CRITERIA	INTERVENTIONS
3 Anxiety *r.t. uncertainty of fetal well-being*	• Verbalizes feelings, fears, concerns at all times	• Encourage expressions of feelings of - ambivalence - fears/concerns • Discuss potential complications of labor and delivery
	• Recognizes relief of stress	• Monitor FHR, VS, BP q4h and prn; share assessment of findings with patient • Give reassurance to feelings of concern regarding high risk status • Refer to SW, pastoral care, peer support group
	• Demonstrates effective coping skills	• Monitor and assess identified coping skills q shift • Identify and assess support system
		RATIONALE: *Information and opportunities to explore concerns will minimize anxiety.*
4 Knowledge Deficit *r.t. pregnancy issues, lack of exposure to problem*	• Verbalizes use, dose, and side effects of medications	• Teach medication purpose, side effects, correct doses, and timing
	• Demonstrates ADL and exercise routines	• Arrange for dietitian to counsel regarding Na restriction • Teach physiological changes as related to pregnancy and disease state • Teach s/s of CHF • Teach use of left lateral recumbent position
		RATIONALE: *Mother has fear of unknown due to lack of knowledge or experience; outcome of pregnancy is closely related to preventative measures.*

OTHER LESS COMMON NURSING DIAGNOSES: *High Risk for Infection; Impaired Gas Exchange; Altered Tissue Perfusion (renal, cardiopulmonary); High Risk for Injury (fetal); Anticipatory Grieving; Impaired Home Maintenance*

ESSENTIAL DISCHARGE CRITERIA

- FHR, fetal movement reassuring
- Shows BP WNL
- Exhibits no dyspnea, no rales
- Identifies plan for bed rest, modified ADL
- Demonstrates successful coping skills
- Affirms need for close medical supervision; verbalizes knowledge of medication administration

CHEMICAL DEPENDENCY

NURSING DIAGNOSES	OUTCOME CRITERIA	INTERVENTIONS
1 Altered Nutrition: Less than body requirements *r.t. body weight 20% or more under ideal, loss of appetite, money spent on drugs rather than food*	• Gains weight (20-25 lb at rate of 1-2 lb/week)	• Teach effects on fetus of low nutrient levels • Weigh daily • Refer to dietitian for counseling • Monitor lab values
	• Demonstrates good diet habits	• Assess eating habits, likes, dislikes, knowledge of nutrition pyramid
		RATIONALE: *Prevent IUGR and other complications to fetus and mother.*
2 High Risk for Infection *r.t. malnutrition, inadequate primary defenses, invasive procedures*	• Verbalizes understanding of prevention techniques	• Teach infection causes and prevention – universal precautions - STD - HIV/AIDS • Monitor cultures, CBC reports • Assess for s/s of infection - temperature, HR q2-4h • Teach potential effects on fetus
		RATIONALE: *Substance abusers have altered perceptions of how their actions may increase the potential for harm.*
3 Altered Tissue Perfusion *r.t. sudden excessive hypertension, vasoconstriction, PTL*	• FHR and activity WNL	• Assess for fetal well-being - FHR - fetal movement - BPP as ordered • Measure fundal height q week
	• Experiences no PTL, irritable uterus	• Discuss effects of substance abuse on fetal well-being • Assess for UC, irritability
		RATIONALE: *Substance abuse creates disturbance in placental fetal circulation, placing the fetus at risk for hypoxia and IUGR.*

NURSING DIAGNOSES	OUTCOME CRITERIA	INTERVENTIONS
4 Self-Esteem Disturbance *r.t. self-destructive behavior, lack of coping skills, domestic/sexual violence*	• Demonstrates positive or improving attitudes toward self	• Establish a trusting relationship; ensure privacy • Encourage truthful disclosure of addiction history • Assess for history of domestic violence and/or sexual abuse • Offer information about the substance and its effect on the fetus • Refer to SW or counseling program
		RATIONALE: *Addiction may be a result of low self-esteem, an escape from the lack of coping skills. Assessment of domestic and/or sexual violence is important since there is an association with chemical abuse.*
5 High Risk for Altered Parenting *r.t. lack of attachment behaviors, addictive behavior*	• Verbalizes expectations, fears, concerns, potential for protective services	• Facilitate verbalization of expectations, fears, concerns, guilt • Assess support system • Refer to SW or community agency
	• Discusses plan for gaining infant care skills	• Refer to "parent friend" or mentoring program to gain caregiving skills • Give explanation of infant's expected withdrawal behaviors • Assess understanding of parental role • Provide educational resources regarding infant care techniques
		RATIONALE: *The addicted person may not be able to focus on the infant if the disease is advanced, or they may lack the skills necessary to demonstrate minimally effective parenting.*

OTHER LESS COMMON NURSING DIAGNOSES: *Family Coping: Potential for Growth; Fear; Knowledge Deficit; Powerlessness; High Risk for Injury (fetal)*

ESSENTIAL DISCHARGE CRITERIA

- Demonstrates weight gain
- Verbalizes/displays behaviors essential to minimize potential for infection
- Verbalizes s/s of PTL and importance of timely call to PCP
- Maintains FHR and activity WNL
- Possesses information and/or appointment for substance abuse support and counseling
- Verbalizes understanding of parameters for protective services involvement

DIABETES MELLITUS

NURSING DIAGNOSES	OUTCOME CRITERIA	INTERVENTIONS
1 High Risk for Fluid Volume Deficit *r.t. nausea, vomiting, osmotic diuresis associated with ketoacidosis*	• Maintains adequate hydration - good skin turgor - moist mucous membranes - absence of polyphagia, polydipsia, or polyuria - normal LOC	• Measure urine output q8h • Maintain I&O • Weigh daily • Assess for nausea and vomiting • Assess mucous membranes, skin turgor, thirst • Offer appealing forms of fluids within dietary requirements: popsicles, snow cones, jello
	• Exhibits no signs of ketoacidosis - no urinary ketones - electrolytes WNL - blood sugar WNL - VS, BP WNL	• Monitor urine for ketones q voiding • Monitor electrolytes • Monitor blood sugar levels before meals and bedtime snack; use blood glucose meter • Assess VS and BP q8h • Observe for evidence of fruity breath or Kussmaul's respirations • Administer insulin per orders; observe for effects, side effects • Maintain balanced regimen of activity, diet, insulin per orders
		RATIONALE: *Frequent monitoring for s/s of dehydration results in early detection/management.*
2 High Risk for Injury *r.t. altered cerebral tissue perfusion (edema) associated with ketoacidosis*	• Exhibits no s/s of cerebral edema - is alert, oriented - has normal pupillary reaction, vision - shows normal gait, demeanor	• Assess LOC and pupillary reactions q1-4h • Assess changes in vision q1-4h • Observe for ataxia, irritability, confusion q1-4h
	• Demonstrates normal VS, BP	• Monitor VS, BP q1-4h as indicated
		RATIONALE: *Frequent assessment of s/s of cerebral edema results in early detection/management of ketoacidosis and prevents the complication of brain damage.*

NURSING DIAGNOSES	OUTCOME CRITERIA	INTERVENTIONS
3 Knowledge Deficit *r.t. unfamiliarity with diagnosis, complex information*	• Discusses s/s, causes, treatment of diabetes mellitus	• Teach about the s/s, treatment, causes of increased blood sugar • Consult educator knowledgeable about diabetes
	• Reiterates correct knowledge of treatment regimen - indications for glucagon - actions of insulin - dose adjustments - rules for sick days - waiting times for meals - when to seek help	• Teach s/s, treatment, causes of decreased blood sugar • Teach the s/s, treatment, causes of ketoacidosis • Identify parameters to call to attention of PCP
		RATIONALE: *Knowledge of the relationship of blood sugar levels, activity, diet, and insulin is basic to successful management of diabetes. Knowledge of s/s of ketoacidosis is essential to prompt requests for assistance from physician or other care provider.*
4 Ineffective Individual Coping *r.t. diabetic management adaptations*	• Verbalize satisfaction with treatment plan	• Encourage expression of feelings, questions • Involve in hospital care regimen • Involve in evaluation of actual hypo/ hyperglycemic episodes
	• Shows agreement, understanding of the care regimen in hospital and at home	• Facilitate home care planning - refer to community support groups - discuss home care situations and help with family anticipatory problem-solving - verify possession of names and numbers of physician, clinic, emergency care facilities - involve home care coordinator in planning
		RATIONALE: *Active involvement in the hospital provides a sense of control and comfort that fosters mastery of the learning and coping skills needed for successful care management at home.*

ANTEPARTUM

OTHER LESS COMMON NURSING DIAGNOSES: *High Risk for Injury (fetus); Altered Nutrition: Greater than body requirements; Noncompliance; High Risk for Infection; Ineffective Management of Therapeutic Regimen*

ESSENTIAL DISCHARGE CRITERIA

- FHR is reactive
- Exhibits no extreme fluctuations in blood sugar
- Has balanced I&O
- Demonstrates correct blood glucose monitoring and urine ketone testing technique
- Verbalizes knowledge of s/s, treatment, causes of hypo- and hyperglycemia
- Demonstrates kick counts and verbalizes when to call PCP
- Possesses identification tag, emergency phone numbers, and follow-up appointments with physician

DOMESTIC VIOLENCE

NURSING DIAGNOSES	OUTCOME CRITERIA	INTERVENTIONS
1 High Risk for Injury *r.t. domestic violence*	• Accepts referral information	• On admission, assess for exposure to domestic violence, ensure privacy - "Do you feel safe in your home" or "Have you ever felt threatened or been harmed by someone close to you?"
	• Acknowledges physical abuse and/or neglect as illegal acts	• Provide "pocket" information card regarding community services • Refer to social services, pastoral care • Realize that patient may not acknowledge domestic violence or openly accept printed information or referral
	• Verbalizes escape plan	• Discuss importance of having an escape plan - place to go, how to get there - take important papers: birth certificate, private papers, bank account number, money - consider hiding packed suitcase, give to friend • Identify leaving as a time of increased risk for harm, need for thorough planning for safety of self and children
	• Shows no s/s of PTL or fetal distress	• Assess for preterm labor - monitor uterine contractions - assess FHR, activity • Teach s/s of PTL and risk of fetal distress secondary to trauma to mother

RATIONALE: *Domestic violence increases during pregnancy. PTL is associated with domestic abuse and/or neglect.*

OTHER LESS COMMON NURSING DIAGNOSES: *Altered Family Process; Ineffective Individual Coping; Self-Esteem Disturbance; Knowledge Deficit*

ESSENTIAL DISCHARGE CRITERIA

- FHR reactive, fetus active
- No PTL or other signs of pregnancy compromise

ECTOPIC PREGNANCY

NURSING DIAGNOSES	OUTCOME CRITERIA	INTERVENTIONS
1 **Pain (acute)** *r.t. abdominal bleeding secondary to rupture of fallopian tube*	• Experiences increasing comfort level - pain scale scores improve - VS stabilize within acceptable ranges - relaxed body posture, facial expression	• Ask patient to rate pain on level of 0-10 (0=no pain; 10=worst pain) • Assess nonverbal cues regarding level of pain • Assess VS to establish baseline • Provide care in an unhurried, supportive manner • Assist to position of most comfort • Allow expression of fears • Administer pain medication after diagnosis is confirmed to avoid masking symptoms • Anticipate need for surgical intervention **RATIONALE:** *Pain is an important diagnostic cue in fallopian tube rupture.*
2 **Knowledge Deficit** *r.t. diagnosis and treatment of ectopic pregnancy*	• Expresses understanding of diagnosis and treatment options	• Explain treatments and procedures prior to implementation • Gear communication to the understanding of patient and family • Involve support person in teaching process • Evaluate and document patient's level of understanding of diagnosis • Assist patient in understanding long-term consequences of condition • Administer RhoGAM to Rh negative women within 72 h **RATIONALE:** *Education decreases fear and leads to better patient cooperation.*

NURSING DIAGNOSES	OUTCOME CRITERIA	INTERVENTIONS
3 Anticipatory Grieving *r.t. pregnancy loss*	• Patient/family expresses feelings regarding loss - participate in grief work - utilize appropriate resources	• Assess patient/family history r.t. loss and coping abilities • Identify existing support systems, refer to appropriate resources • Encourage patient/family to express feelings • Inform patient/family of grieving process • Respect culture, religions, race, and values of patient/family as they express grief **RATIONALE:** *Grief work is important in resolving the pregnancy loss.*

OTHER LESS COMMON NURSING DIAGNOSIS: *Fluid Volume Deficit; Fear; Ineffective Coping*

ESSENTIAL DISCHARGE CRITERIA

- VS WNL
- Shows Hb and Hct and clotting factors WNL
- Reports increased level of comfort
- Verbalizes understanding of condition and s/s of recurrence
- Identifies available community resources for grief work and potential infertility problems

GENITAL/VAGINAL TRACT INFECTION

NURSING DIAGNOSES	OUTCOME CRITERIA	INTERVENTIONS

See "Infectious Disorders" care plan in Antepartal Section

NURSING DIAGNOSES	OUTCOME CRITERIA	INTERVENTIONS
1 Impaired Skin Integrity *r.t. invasion of infectious organisms*	• Heals without complications	• Assess perineum for blisters, ulcers, warts, or signs of infection • Note color, odor, and consistency of drainage • Document patient history of STD, diabetes, antibiotic therapy, or immunologic suppression • Promote hydration • Promote dry/clean healing environment • Discuss appropriate dietary implications **RATIONALE:** *These measures promote healing by enhancing self-care capabilities.*
2 Pain (acute) *r.t. s/s of infection*	• Reports an increase in comfort level	• Assess patient's level of discomfort on a scale 0-10 (0=no pain; 10=worst pain) • Assess nonverbal cues indicative of pain • Assist patient to use relaxation techniques during perineal/pelvic exams and cultures • Assess comfort measures utilized by the patient • Provide emotional support when assisting in diagnosis/evaluation of patient's condition **RATIONALE:** *Promote comfort and enhance self-care capabilities.*

NURSING DIAGNOSES	OUTCOME CRITERIA	INTERVENTIONS
3 Knowledge Deficit *r.t. treatment, prevention of genital/vaginal tract infection*	• Expresses understanding of diagnosis, treatment, and prevention of genital/vaginal infections	• Assist in identification of predisposing factors r.t. infection • Evaluate patient's knowledge of condition • Use a multidisciplinary approach to assure continuity of care • Explain treatments and procedures prior to implementation • Communicate on the patient's level using a nonjudgmental attitude
	• Affirms need to seek early treatment of subsequent infections	• Assist patient in understanding the importance of prevention, early detection, and treatment of infections • Assist understanding of potential long-term consequences of genital/vaginal infections • Identify appropriate community resources
		RATIONALE: *Education promotes early treatment and prevention of infections and may help prevent serious complications.*

OTHER LESS COMMON NURSING DIAGNOSIS: *Altered Urinary Elimination; Anxiety; Altered Sexuality Patterns; High Risk for Injury (fetal)*

ESSENTIAL DISCHARGE CRITERIA

- Shows no evidence of genital/vaginal tract infection
- Lab studies/cultures WNL
- Expresses increased comfort
- FHR reactive
- Expresses knowledge of condition and prevention measures
- Identifies, affirms use of appropriate community resources

HERPES SIMPLEX VIRUS

NURSING DIAGNOSES	OUTCOME CRITERIA	INTERVENTIONS
1 Knowledge Deficit *r.t. etiology, disease process, treatment and outcome of disease*	• Verbalizes understanding of HSV, treatment, prevention of spread, isolation	• Provide information on transmission of HSV, s/s of infection, treatment protocols, and long-term effects of diseases • Instruct on isolation techniques and institute universal precautions
	• Discusses screening and ongoing follow-up plan	• Educate on importance of having ongoing screening/diagnostic tests to determine activity or inactivity of virus and recognition of any complications • Alert patient of need, at 36 weeks of gestation, to obtain the following tests on a weekly basis - PAP test of lesions - serial antibody titre - viral culture of lesions • Teach patient the importance of reporting to the hospital promptly after membranes rupture • Refer patient to American Social Health Association (has a program run by the Herpes Resource Center which provides a quarterly newsletter and hotline and organizes local self-help groups. Address: P.O. Box 110, Palo Alto, CA 94302).
		RATIONALE: *Patient/significant other must understand the infectious process to lessen risk of spread and facilitate care for family and self.*
2 High Risk for Infection (neonate) *r.t. maternal transmission* *(Refer to "Infectious Disorders" care plan)*	• Infant shows no signs of HSV infection - VS WNL - breath sounds clear, equal bilaterally - no apnea - no lethargy or poor feeding - culture negative	• Observe and screen infant for symptoms of sepsis, metabolic disturbances, conjunctivitis, jaundice, respiratory distress, convulsions, and other neurologic involvement - culture of mucous membranes at 24-48h of birth - VS q4-8h, skin color at each feeding and q4h • Auscultate chest q4-8h in supine and upright positions • Monitor blood glucose q4-8h

NURSING DIAGNOSES	OUTCOME CRITERIA	INTERVENTIONS
		• Monitor blood glucose q4-8h • Instruct patient on infant care; the importance of follow-up by pediatrician
		RATIONALE: *Diligent assessment and observation facilitates prompt recognition of presence of infection.*
3 Pain *r.t. presence of vesicular lesions on cervix, vagina, and/or vulva*	• Verbalizes decreased pain	• Administer prescribed analgesics as indicated
	• Shows dry and healing vesicles	• Apply warm soaks with solutions such as boric acid or Epsom salts to promote healing and drying • Use drying agents such as alcohol and local heat to hasten healing of lesions. *No* ointments, salves, topical ether, or bacillus Calmette-Guérin vaccination
		RATIONALE: *Aiding the drying of vesicles decreases shedding which is the primary mode of HSV spread.*
4 Anxiety *r.t. maternal injury from HSV*	• VS WNL	• Monitor VS q4-8h as prescribed
	• Identifies s/s for prompt recognition of infection	• Observe for s/s of infection - fever, malaise - anorexia, local - lymphadenopathy - dysuria, urinary - retention
	• Demonstrates stress reduction	• Emphasize stress reduction techniques to lessen risk of recurrence
		RATIONALE: *Lessen risk of recurrence and/or recognize complications and treat appropriately to help prevent sequelae.*

ANTEPARTUM

OTHER LESS COMMON NURSING DIAGNOSES:
Impaired Skin Integrity; High Risk for Injury (fetal)

ESSENTIAL DISCHARGE CRITERIA

- Afebrile
- Lesions healing
- FHR WNL, fetus active
- Demonstrates knowledge regarding self and fetus related to HSV and s/s to report to PCP immediately
- Verbalizes importance of follow-up appointments for self

NURSING DIAGNOSES	OUTCOME CRITERIA	INTERVENTIONS
1 Knowledge Deficit *r.t. lack of information about the disease process, mode of transmission, complications, treatment, and continuing healthcare*	• Identifies s/s of infection and precautions to avoid transmission	• Review the s/s of infection; explain disease process and methods of preventing HIV transmission • Teach patient/partner how to check for s/s of opportunistic infections and cancer
	• Verbalizes knowledge of s/s to report to physician	• Teach s/s to report to physician • Provide information about early manifestations of HIV infection - fatigue - oral thrush - night sweats - fever and other flulike symptoms - vaginal infections
	• Discusses treatment regimen	• Instruct about importance of having follow-up screening and/or diagnostic tests and gynecologic evaluations (both ante- and postpartum) - HIV/AIDS test - Pap smear (cervical and anal) with colposcopic examination - disseminated infections such as CMV, herpes, *Candida*
	• Reiterates knowledge of medications: dosage, route of administration, schedule, effects, side effects	• Teach about prescribed medications, purpose, names, dosage, time of administration, toxic side effects to be reported
	• Affirms knowledge of follow-up appointments	• Explain importance of follow-up appointments with all care providers and laboratory
	• Describes own needs for support and identifies resources specific to those needs	• Provide information about resources that may assist in coping with disease - community AIDS hotlines - psychological resources - social services - resources for financial assistance
	• Participates in discussion about partner's need for testing	• Assist the patient in preparing to inform husband/partner of infection and any tests and/or treatment he/she may need

NURSING DIAGNOSES	OUTCOME CRITERIA	INTERVENTIONS
	• Verbalizes knowledge of prevention of disease	• Teach how to prevent spread of infection - discuss risk factors; advise "safe sex" practices; advise to not share personal items such as toothbrushes, razors - discuss results of HIV tests (ELISA, Western blot, etc.) - discuss potential for newborn to convert to HIV positive - listen to concerns; assist to problem-solve lifestyle issues
		RATIONALE: *Both patient and partner must understand the disease process so they can care for her and the family without transmitting the infection to them.*
2 High Risk for Infection *r.t. depressed immune system* *(Refer to "Infectious Disorders" care plan)*	• Verbalizes understanding of and complies with universal precautions	• Explain isolation precautions necessary by the health team to prevent spread of infection • Explain and institute universal precautions as per CDC
	• Experiences early detection of the s/s of infection	• Monitor VS, BP q4h; record temperature more frequently if trending beginning
	• Experiences prompt treatment for infection - balanced I&O - no frequency, burning on urination - urine clear, amber - clear breath sounds - no thick, yellow sputum - normal VS	• Explain need to report s/s of infection to care provider • Monitor I&O; report urinary frequency, burning, or changes in character of urine • Monitor and report changes in breath sounds, increase in RR/rhythm, any cough, and change in sputum • Use aseptic/antiseptic techniques for all invasive procedures: IV site(s), vaginal/rectal exam • Administer medications as ordered; assess response, report side effects

NURSING DIAGNOSES	OUTCOME CRITERIA	INTERVENTIONS
	• Achieves normal or normalizing lab values, per orders	• Monitor lab data daily or as prescribed - CBC with differential, platelet count - type, Rh, and antibody screening - rubella titer, HbsAg - purified protein derivative - T-cell count - GC, VDRL, TORCH - BUN, creatinine - liver enzymes - total protein - x-ray
		RATIONALE: *Treatment and monitoring control the current infection and enable prompt recognition and treatment of other opportunistic infections.*
3 High Risk for Injury (fetal and neonatal) *r.t. transmission of HIV*	• Gravida/partner discuss significance of all tests	• Explain the meaning of passive and active immunity and implications on the fetus/neonate • Obtain antepartum fetal surveillance tests as ordered • Be prepared to provide high risk care to neonate as necessary - communicate with neonatal caregivers
	• Verbalizes understanding of appropriate infection control practices which allow interaction with the neonate	• Teach patient how to prevent spread of infection to newborn
	• Understands results of the antepartum test (to allow for informed decision-making)	• Counsel regarding breastfeeding and support decision • Encourage mother/infant bonding, while reinforcing isolation practices
	• Patient/partner discuss need for limiting pregnancy in future; for lifestyle changes; need for medical follow-up	• Facilitate decision-making - discuss potential for infected infant in subsequent pregnancies - offer referral to family planning services - encourage constant medical supervision - verify follow-up appointments

NURSING DIAGNOSES	OUTCOME CRITERIA	INTERVENTIONS
		RATIONALE: *Treatment protects the infant from any sequelae from maternal infection. Monitoring detects any spread of infection, enabling prompt treatment.*
4 Altered Sexuality Patterns *r.t. potential for disease transmission, fear of rejection by husband/partner and depressed libido*	• Verbalizes understanding of how HIV is spread	• Determine knowledge of and attitudes about AIDS in relation to sexuality • Provide forum for expressions of anger, anxiety, and concerns
	• Identifies safe sexual practices • Expresses commitment to safe behavior	• Explain safe-sex guidelines and practices
	• Makes positive statements concerning alternate modes of sexual expression	• Encourage couple to focus on the strengths of their relationship and encourage dialogue of their concerns and feelings • Be nonjudgmental and explain normalcy of feelings expressed • Provide information on alternate methods of sexual expression while avoiding activities that permit exchange of body fluid (feces or blood) between partners
		RATIONALE: *Knowledge of safe practices enables patient and partner to enjoy a physically and emotionally satisfying sexual/intimate experience without spreading HIV.*
5 Social Isolation *r.t. grief, stigma of illness, powerlessness over prognosis, and loss of further childbearing potential*	• Continues social interaction with family and partner	• Monitor for s/s of dysfunctional grief and initiate referrals for counseling
	• Makes positive comments about self and about support of significant other, family, and friends	• Discuss and support personal strengths and coping mechanisms • Encourage visits with friends and significant others

NURSING DIAGNOSES	OUTCOME CRITERIA	INTERVENTIONS
		RATIONALE: *Facilitate progress through the grieving process using effective coping mechanisms with partner and family support.*
6 High Risk for Impaired Skin Integrity *r.t. lesions and infections associated with depressed immune system*	• Has clear, intact skin	• Provide and encourage skin care q4-8h and after elimination • Clean skin lesions with soap and water and prescribed ointment
	• Reports skin free of itching, dryness	• Inspect skin q8h and document changes
		RATIONALE: *Skin and tissue remain free of new areas of excoriation and breakdown when good skin care is provided.*
7 Altered Nutrition: Less than body requirements *r.t. anorexia, nausea, vomiting, stomatitis, malabsorption*	• Takes 80% of prescribed diet at each meal	• Change eating patterns to increase appetite - small, frequent meals - light meals - serve dry, bland, cool foods and fluids • Provide antinausea medications half hour before eating • Provide high-protein, high-calorie supplements • Provide high-calorie fruits, vegetables, and main dishes • Consult with nutritionist to plan diet
	• Reports throat and esophagus not sore	• Administer oral hygiene before and after meals
	• Shows normalizing lab values	• Monitor electrolytes, serum albumin, and total protein daily or as prescribed
	• Shows body weight increasing or stabilizing	• Weigh daily • Notify PCP when intake and output are not equivalent and/or weight decreased by 3-5%

NURSING DIAGNOSES	OUTCOME CRITERIA	INTERVENTIONS
		RATIONALE: *These nursing measures help to supply the body with the required nutritional demands; decrease metabolic demands to facilitate the action of the immune system.*

OTHER LESS COMMON NURSING DIAGNOSES: *Body Image Disturbance; Situational Low Self-Esteem; Ineffective Management of Therapeutic Regimen; Impaired Home Maintenance Management*

ESSENTIAL DISCHARGE CRITERIA

- Is afebrile
- Shows stable or increasing body weight
- All family members have HIV and other required tests completed as indicated
- FHR reactive
- Patient and partner discuss need for family planning services, early and meticulous prenatal care for subsequent pregnancies
- Referrals are made to social services, counseling as indicated

HYPEREMESIS GRAVIDARUM

NURSING DIAGNOSES	OUTCOME CRITERIA	INTERVENTIONS
1 High Risk for Fluid Volume Deficit *r.t. protracted nausea, vomiting*	• Exhibits normal VS, serum electrolytes, Hb, Hct	• Monitor VS, lab values q4h; report abnormalities
	• Maintains balanced I&O	• Maintain strict I&O
	• Has urinary output > 30 mL/h - normal sp. gr. - negative for ketones	• Measure output; test urinary sp. gr. and ketones q4-8h
	• Shows good skin turgor, moist mucous membranes	• Inspect skin, mucous membranes q8h
	• Denies syncope, vertigo, malaise	• Query regarding dizziness, faintness, malaise q8h
	• Tolerates diet advances; takes > 1800 cal/day	• Provide ordered nutrition, fluids - offer small, frequent meals, preferred fluids; advance as tolerated - encourage increasing fluids in small amounts throughout day
		RATIONALE: *Careful dietary and fluid intake reduces vomiting. Monitoring of hydration prompts timely interventions to increase fluid intake.*
2 Altered Nutrition: Less than body requirements *r.t. protracted nausea, vomiting*	• Shows normal weight gain for trimester	• Weigh daily • Inspect ankles, hands, face for edema bid (edema may mask real weight gain, loss)
	• Does not guard abdomen • Has normal bowel sounds	• Monitor for distention bid; report abnormalities - inspect abdomen for contour changes, tenderness - auscultate bowel sounds
	• Takes 80% of prescribed foods, fluids	• Assess emesis: time, duration, amount, characteristics, relationship to intake, precipitating or relieving factors • Encourage small meals throughout day

NURSING DIAGNOSES	OUTCOME CRITERIA	INTERVENTIONS
	• Makes proper food choices for balanced diet	• Assess and plan diet - maintain food diary: what, how much taken and retained, how prepared - minimize fat intake • Consult dietitian • Administer antinausea medications per orders; assess effects
		RATIONALE: *Appropriate weight gain is consistent with adequate food intake. Assessing bowel sounds helps to rule out obstruction as cause of vomiting. Careful dietary and fluid intake reduces nausea and promotes adequate nutrition.*
3 Pain (chronic) *r.t. gastric distress associated with protracted vomiting*	• Reports reasonable comfort, relief from nausea	• Keep leftover food, other odors away • Maintain cool, calm environment • Provide oral hygiene before and after each snack and meal and after each emesis • Maintain in high Fowler's or upright for 30 min after food, fluid intake to minimize discomfort
	• Identifies methods for counteracting nausea	• Involve patient in own nausea control for management at home
		RATIONALE: *Managing the environment and encouraging good oral hygiene maximizes food retention and minimizes discomfort.*
4 Anxiety *r.t. the fear of loss of pregnancy, loss of control*	• Verbalizes anxiety and identifies means to relieve stress	• Encourage patient to ask questions • Teach relaxation techniques • Counsel about need to identify stressors and how to avoid them • Assess support system and refer to community agencies as necessary • Encourage verbalization of feelings regarding pregnancy and/or illness
		RATIONALE: *Verbalization of fears and identification of stressors reduces anxiety.*

NURSING DIAGNOSES	OUTCOME CRITERIA	INTERVENTIONS
5 **Knowledge Deficit** *r.t. lack of understanding of management of vomiting, nutrition*	• Discusses disease process, treatment rationale; asks appropriate questions	• Explain disease process, rationale for treatment, expected course of recovery
	• Selects required nutrients from list • Discusses methods of controlling nausea	• Assist in planning diet - review required nutrients - discuss ways to decrease nausea, vomiting - involve patient in selecting and evaluating food intake and in nausea control
	• Performs urine ketone test	• Show how to test for ketones
	• Lists reportable s/s: edema, dizziness, ketonuria	• Describe reportable s/s and their significance
	• Verbalizes fears about pregnancy, health of infant; includes partner in discussions if appropriate	• Explain potential for low birth weight infant; listen to concerns
	• Identifies support system	• Assist in finding support system

RATIONALE: *Since the patient will be managing the problem at home, she needs to discover the best methods for diet and nausea management.*

OTHER LESS COMMON NURSING DIAGNOSES: *Constipation; Social Isolation; Ineffective Individual Coping; Impaired Home Maintenance Management*

ESSENTIAL DISCHARGE CRITERIA

- Tolerates fluids and eating small meals
- Demonstrates at least one relaxation method
- Verbalizes understanding of nutrition/fluid requirements
- Identifies support systems and plans for follow-up

ERTENSION, PREGNANCY INDUCED

NURSING DIAGNOSES	OUTCOME CRITERIA	INTERVENTIONS
1 High Risk for Injury (maternal) *r.t. increased arterial pressure, decreased renal perfusion, cyclic vasospasm, cerebral edema*	• Shows BP WNL	• Monitor BP, report as indicated (> 140/90 mmHg, systolic rise > 30 mmHg, or diastolic rise > 15 mmHg over baseline) • Administer antihypertensives as ordered
	• Maintains fluid balance and adequate urine output	• Monitor I&O • Measure urine protein using testing strip method • Obtain daily weights • Assess for edema
	• Exhibits no symptoms of CNS involvement (headaches, seizures, visual disturbances, hyperreflexia)	• Keep on bed rest in left lateral position as prescribed • Assess CNS q4-8h
	• Shows no s/s $MgSO_4$ toxicity	• Administer $MgSO_4$, monitor blood levels as ordered - RR > 12/min - DTR present - no LOC
	• Takes prescribed diet • Verbalizes knowledge of diet and its rationale • Selects correct foods from list	• Provide and instruct about a high protein and low Na diet or diet as prescribed; consult dietitian
		RATIONALE: *Increasing BP, edema, weight gain, and proteinuria are symptoms of worsening preeclampsia; bed rest in the left lateral position increases uteroplacental blood flow and perfusion of the kidneys and diuresis and is beneficial in helping to lower the BP. A low Na, high protein diet reduces fluid retention and aids diuresis.*
2 High Risk for Injury (fetal) *r.t. decreased uteroplacental perfusion, hypoxia, premature birth, and abruptio placentae*	• Delivers healthy infant at term • Verbalizes no decrease in fetal activity	• Assess FHR and activity q1-4h as ordered

NURSING DIAGNOSES	OUTCOME CRITERIA	INTERVENTIONS
	• Verbalizes understanding of need to seek immediate medical attention for decreased fetal kick counts and s/s of preterm labor or abruptio placentae	• Teach patient fetal movement counts • Teach patient to recognize s/s of premature labor and abruptio placentae
		RATIONALE: *Daily fetal kick counts are indicators of fetal well-being. Patient's ability to recognize the symptoms of PTL can enable her to obtain medical care in time to delay delivery if needed. Abruptio placentae is a life-threatening complication of preeclampsia, and patients need to know when to obtain immediate medical care .*
3 Excess Fluid Volume *r.t. fluid retention, decreased renal blood flow, decreased GFR*	• Shows urine output > 30 mL/h - protein ≤ trace - sp. gr. WNL	• Monitor I&O qh; anticipate need for urinary catheter
	• Shows intake of 100-125 mL/h	• Closely monitor IV fluid administration - place on infusion pump • Calculate total fluid intake; discuss with patient how to divide oral intake allotment across 24h period
	• Shows no edema - skin dry, intact	• Assess feet, legs, hands, face for edema - minimize potential for skin breakdown
	• Breath sounds clear, equal bilaterally	• Auscultate breath sounds q2-4h as indicated • Administer O_2 as ordered • Elevate HOB for SOB • Provide BSC to minimize exertion
		RATIONALE: *Fluid retention and/or fluid overload needs close observation to delineate cause/effect, thereby guiding appropriate interventions.*

NURSING DIAGNOSES	OUTCOME CRITERIA	INTERVENTIONS
4 Fear *r.t. risk of harm to self and fetus*	• Reports a decrease in level of anxiety and fear	• Allow patient to verbalize her fears and anxiety
	• Family mobilizes in support of patient and her plan of care	• Teach patient and family about PIH and rationale for interventions • Involve family in care of patient to improve her ability to maintain bed rest • Reassure patient as to fetal well-being when appropriate
		RATIONALE: *Verbalizing anxiety and fears can help to relieve them by allowing the patient to express both real and imagined concerns. Teaching about the disease process and how to cooperate with the treatment plan helps relieve anxiety and gives the patient some control over her own health status. Mobilizing the family to be supportive relieves anxiety.*

OTHER LESS COMMON NURSING DIAGNOSES: *Altered Tissue Perfusion (cardiopulmonary, cerebral); Diversional Activity Deficit; Impaired Gas Exchange; Decreased Cardiac Output; High Risk for Infection; High Risk for Impaired Skin Integrity; Knowledge Deficit*

ESSENTIAL DISCHARGE CRITERIA

- Exhibits decreasing, normalizing BP
- Gains < 1 lb/week
- Shows resolving edema
- Urine output WNL, protein trace
- Fetal active, FHR WNL for gestation
- Verbalizes plan for home care, follow-up, support services in place

INFECTIOUS DISORDERS

NURSING DIAGNOSES	OUTCOME CRITERIA	INTERVENTIONS
1 Altered Health Maintenance *r.t. lack of prevention of transmission of infection*	• Follows agreed-upon plan to maintain health	• Encourage to share feelings about change in health status and effects on life • Observe and augment knowledge of disease, treatment, and capacity to follow the treatment regimen • Assist in organizing change in healthcare plan into daily life (i.e., when to take pills, etc.) • Instruct patient/family in treatment regimen: medications, changes of ADLs, how to cope, s/s of reinfection, dietary changes, when to call care provider • Refer to social services for information on community resources (financial, support groups, agencies) • Refer client to community agencies for follow-up care • Verify that follow-up appointments are made prior to discharge; verify how client will be able to attend appointments
		RATIONALE: *When clients participate and agree on the healthcare plan, they are more likely to follow the plan.*
2 High Risk for Infection (transmission to others) *r.t. contagious organisms*	• Is free of s/s of infection - no erythema, localized warmth - no purulent discharges - normal body temperature	• Monitor for symptoms of infection: redness, warmth, discharge, and elevated body temperature q2-6h • Utilize universal precautions
	• Has normal WBC count and differential	• Monitor laboratory values (WBC, differential, serum albumin, serum protein, and cultures)
	• Describes symptoms of infection	• Teach patient how to recognize s/s of infection
	• Demonstrates proper handwashing, oral care, and perineal care	• Teach and encourage correct hygiene - handwashing - oral care - perineal care • Encourage rest periods

NURSING DIAGNOSES	OUTCOME CRITERIA	INTERVENTIONS
		• Use sterile technique performing invasive monitoring • Instruct and reinforce need to practice safe sex as indicated
		RATIONALE: *Increasing the client's awareness of the transmission process helps him or her recognize the s/s of the infection and the need to break the transmission cycle.*
3 Social Isolation *r.t. infectious disease*	• Initiates interactions with others; sets and meets goals	• Encourage social interaction as possible within consideration of physical status • Work one-on-one with client: - build trusting relationship - listen attentively - offer support
	• Identifies reason for feelings of isolation	• Discuss causes of isolation: disease, fear • Encourage patient/family to contact support groups
		RATIONALE: *Providing support, listening attentively, and building a relationship enables the client to take control and responsibility for infection control.*

OTHER LESS COMMON NURSING DIAGNOSES: *Fatigue; Activity Intolerance; Ineffective Individual Coping; Pain; Diarrhea; Altered Urinary Elimination; High Risk for Injury (fetus)*

ESSENTIAL DISCHARGE CRITERIA

- FHR and activity WNL
- Describes specific plan for infection prevention, control, and follow-up
- Describes, demonstrates required infection control techniques: handwashing, oral care, perineal care
- Verbalizes confidence in ability to initiate safe interactions with others
- Describes s/s to report to PCP

ISOIMMUNE DISEASE

NURSING DIAGNOSES	OUTCOME CRITERIA	INTERVENTIONS
1 High Risk for Injury (fetal) *r.t. hemolytic effects of maternal antibodies*	• Indirect Coombs' test negative on first visit and at 28 weeks gestation	• Assess for history of potential past sensitization, such as previous pregnancy, amniocentesis, abortion, or transfusions • Assess father's blood type and Rh factor if mother is Rh negative
	• Antibody titre remains < 1:4 throughout the pregnancy	• Monitor lab values - repeat indirect Coombs' at 28 weeks - report to PCP as indicated - if Rh titre > 1:8, anticipate need for ultrasound and amniocentesis for optical density analysis; schedule as directed
	• Experiences prompt detection of - abnormal sized fetal heart - ascites - subcutaneous edema - hydramnios	• Discuss purpose of ultrasonography • Provide opportunity to ventilate concerns
	• Shows negative (or weakly positive) direct Coombs' test on cord blood due to previous administration of immune globulin at 28 weeks gestation	• Administer one dose prophylactic immune globulin at 28 weeks gestation as ordered • If pregnancy terminates before 13 weeks gestation due to gestational trophoblastic disease, abortion, or ectopic pregnancy, administer one dose of immune globulin within 3h as ordered • At or beyond week 13 or after amniocentesis, administer one dose immune globulin as ordered • Administer one dose immune globulin as ordered within 72h after delivery

RATIONALE: *Immune globulin prevents sensitization of Rh negative to Rh positive fetal cells.*

NURSING DIAGNOSES	OUTCOME CRITERIA	INTERVENTIONS
2 Knowledge Deficit *r.t. unfamiliarity with situation*	• Verbalizes understanding of need for periodic testing during pregnancy and administration of immune globulin	• Assess current knowledge level of Rh negative woman regarding isoimmunization and treatment • Discuss/explain pathophysiology of Rh isoimmunization and rationale for periodic antibody titres during pregnancy • Explain purpose of and schedule for administering RhoGAM immune globulin • Encourage verbalization of any concerns and questions
	• Complies with recommended diagnostic and treatment regimen	• Explain any anticipated procedures (amniocentesis, intrauterine transfusion)
		RATIONALE: *Accurate, timely information can reduce maternal (family) anxiety and empower decision-making.*

OTHER LESS COMMON NURSING DIAGNOSES: *Anxiety; Fear; Ineffective Individual Coping; High Risk for Injury (maternal), Anticipatory Grieving*

ESSENTIAL DISCHARGE CRITERIA

- Is physiologically stable: maternal titre < 1:16; spectrophotometric zone A (not B or C); reactive NST or BPP > 8
- FHR and activity WNL
- Receives immune globulin according to protocol, orders
- Delivers viable infant (Intrapartal)
- Verbalizes plan for follow-up and lists s/s to report to PCP

MULTIPLE GESTATION

NURSING DIAGNOSES	OUTCOME CRITERIA	INTERVENTIONS
1 Altered Nutrition: Less than body requirements *r.t. inadequate intake of nutrients in diet*	• Consumes a well-balanced, high calorie diet (2,400 cal/day)	• Increase patient's caloric intake to support growth and development of multiple gestation • Ensure dietary supplements available and taken as indicated
	• Has weight gain that is appropriate throughout pregnancy	• Provide nutritional consult • Weigh weekly • Encourage small frequent meals (4-6 per day) • Help patient to identify food preferences, including foods high in carbohydrates and protein • Outline dietary plan for patient • Increase rest periods • Identify causes of inadequate nutritional intake (decreased appetite, nausea, vomiting, activity, food preferences, beliefs)
		RATIONALE: *A multiple gestation pregnancy requires an increase in calories, protein, minerals (iron), and folic acid to supply the increased fetal and placental mass.*
2 High Risk for Altered Parenting *r.t. delivery of more than one infant*	• Verbalizes level of knowledge and skill to care for infants	• Provide teaching at every opportunity • Assess knowledge and skills of patient about infant care
	• Discusses concerns about parenting role	• Explore patient's specific concerns about parenting • Discuss components of NICU care as appropriate
	• Identifies resources available	• Provide a list of resources and services available • Discuss aspects of newborn infant care • Give information on multiple gestation support group
		RATIONALE: *Multiple births can place an increased demand on the patient's time. A well-educated and supported patient is better able to cope with the stresses of parenting.*

NURSING DIAGNOSES	OUTCOME CRITERIA	INTERVENTIONS
3 Knowledge Deficit *r.t. high risk pregnancy*	• Identifies s/s of premature labor	• Explain s/s of premature labor - uterine cramping, contractions - pelvic pain/pressure - bloody show - change in amount or character of vaginal discharge - nausea/vomiting or diarrhea - back cramping - rupture of membranes - "just don't feel right"
	• Identifies s/s of complications of pregnancy	• Explain s/s of complications of pregnancy - excessive weight gain - proteinuria - nondependent edema - vaginal bleeding - decreased fetal movement • Teach self-palpation of UCs, fetal movement counts • Instruct patient to lie on left side to maximize blood flow to the uterus • Discuss antepartal testing - NST - BPP - amniocentesis - serial ultrasounds
	• Performs self-care activities as appropriate	• Encourage to read educational materials about multiple gestation • Encourage to arrange a schedule for self-care activities; identify plans for assistance at home

RATIONALE: *A high risk pregnancy such as multiple gestation leads to opportunities for education. This patient will have many topics that need to be addressed to reassure her that the pregnancy will have a good outcome.*

NURSING DIAGNOSES	OUTCOME CRITERIA	INTERVENTIONS
4 **Anxiety** *r.t. high risk pregnancy*	• Relates feelings of anxiety about high risk pregnancy; asks questions, seeks clarification	• Tour NICU if possible to prepare for intensive care environment • Assist in identifying support systems and services • Encourage verbalization of concerns about high risk pregnancy • Explain all procedures and support system • Reassure patient that she is taking appropriate actions to maintain pregnancy • Assist with discovering effective coping strategies
		RATIONALE: *A decrease in anxiety will allow the patient to have more control over her pregnancy and will reassure her about the pregnancy outcome.*

OTHER LESS COMMON NURSING DIAGNOSES: *Stress Incontinence; Constipation; High Risk for Activity Intolerance; Altered Sexuality Patterns; Fatigue; Altered Family Processes; Impaired Home Maintenance Management*

ESSENTIAL DISCHARGE CRITERIA

- FHR and activity WNL
- Understands how to support pregnancy with appropriate diet and nutritional intake
- Develops specific coping strategies
- Verbalizes s/s to report to the physician: PTL symptoms, PIH symptoms, bleeding, decreased fetal movement
- Is able to state her feelings about the pregnancy and the possibility that complications may arise

PLACENTA PREVIA

NURSING DIAGNOSES	OUTCOME CRITERIA	INTERVENTIONS
1 High Risk for Injury (fetal) *r.t. decreased placental perfusion*	• FHR remains between 120-160	• Monitor FHR using continuous EFM
	• FHR reactive	• Assess FHR and response to fetal activity continuously • Perform NST as indicated
	• Fetal BPP ≥ 8	• Prepare patient for ultrasound and NST • Document maternal and fetal events during testing
		RATIONALE: *Fetal assessment is an imperative intervention and will guide decisions regarding delivery method.*
2 High Risk for Fluid Volume Deficit *r.t. blood loss*	• Fluid volume maintained	• Monitor patient for bleeding • Note quantity, color, time of onset, and precipitating factors associated with bleeding
	• VS WNL	• Assess VS q15 min until stable; then as condition requires
	• Coagulation profile WNL - Hct > 30%	• Facilitate drawing of lab values; monitor results • Implement measures to prevent bleeding - implement and maintain strict bed rest - avoid enemas, vaginal or rectal exams - place in semi-Fowler's position
	• Is alert, oriented to time, place, and person	• Assess LOC as indicated
	• Urinary output > 30 mL/h	• Monitor urinary output hourly; report oliguria to PCP • Replace fluids, electrolytes, and blood as ordered
		RATIONALE: *Placenta previa places the woman at risk for excessive blood loss and circulatory collapse.*

NURSING DIAGNOSES	OUTCOME CRITERIA	INTERVENTIONS
3 Fear *r.t. threat to self and fetus*	• Verbalizes why she is afraid - expresses feelings	• Encourage patient to verbalize fears • Provide frequent verbal and nonverbal reassurances that may assist in reducing fear • Provide continuity of care through patient assignment • Provide information as necessary
		RATIONALE: *Placenta previa increases the risk of fetal compromise.*
4 Knowledge Deficit *r.t. condition and unanticipated cesarean delivery*	• Verbalizes understanding of condition	• Teach patient about condition and potential problems
	• Expresses understanding of operative delivery process	• Prepare the patient and family for the possibility of surgical intervention
		RATIONALE: *Information will reduce maternal stress and assist with decision-making.*

OTHER LESS COMMON NURSING DIAGNOSES: *Anxiety; Knowledge Deficit; Altered Family Process; Anticipatory Grieving; High Risk for Infection; Altered Tissue Perfusion*

ESSENTIAL DISCHARGE CRITERIA

- FHR remains stable without signs of stress
- Fluid volume remains WNL
- VS WNL
- Verbalizes understanding of s/s to report to PCP immediately

PRETERM LABOR

NURSING DIAGNOSES	OUTCOME CRITERIA	INTERVENTIONS
1 **Pain** *r.t. uterine contractions*	• Positions self in lateral recumbent position	• Discuss importance of maximizing uterine blood flow • Support position with pillows • Place water, telephone, diversional activities within easy reach
	• Experiences no UC	• Assess strength, duration and frequency of UC • Utilize EFM as ordered • Administer tocolytic agents as ordered - $MgSO_4$ - terbutaline sulfate - indomethacin
	• Shows no further cervical dilation	• Assess cervical dilation per physician order
		RATIONALE: *Preterm UC seem to be associated with contracted plasma volume, prolonged physical activity, or irritable uterus.*
2 **Anxiety** *r.t. unknown pregnancy outcome, viability of fetus*	• Displays decreased anxiety	• Facilitate discussion of fears, concerns • Involve support persons
	• Verbalizes realistic plans for the pregnancy	• Provide tour of NICU as indicated • Discuss potential outcome scenarios given the clinical picture; assist in dealing with ambiguity of outcome expectations • Provide written information regarding PTL, delivery, neonatal problems at current gestation
		RATIONALE: *Information provided to meet the patient's and family's concerns offers specific framework for the family to use in coping with PTL.*

NURSING DIAGNOSES	OUTCOME CRITERIA	INTERVENTIONS
3 **Knowledge Deficit** *r.t. inexperience with PTL*	• Identifies, has list of s/s of PTL	• Discuss s/s of PTL to report to nurse/PCP • Provide printed materials to reinforce teaching • Document discharge teaching thoroughly
	• Demonstrates uterine palpation technique	• Demonstrate uterine palpation • Discuss assessment and recording of contractions at home • Provide with written follow-up plan, phone numbers
	• Describes, demonstrates self-care strategies to minimize the potential for PTL	• Discuss strategies to decrease potential for PTL - drink at least 8-10 glasses of fluids daily - pace activities to minimize fatigue - avoid prolonged standing - when sitting or lying down, tilt to side/lie on side - call PCP at earliest sign of contractions • Refer to preterm birth prevention program for telephone follow-up
		RATIONALE: *Prompt detection of PTL and early intervention will potentially prevent cervical dilation.*
4 **Caregiver Role Strain** *r.t. bed rest, lack of support for self-care, child care, and home maintenance management*	• Describes plan for self-care at home	• Discuss strategies for self-care given bed rest limitations - cooler at bedside/couch filled with juices, snacks, sandwich - position phone, radio, TV, reading material within easy reach - if stairs in the home, set up self-care area on same floor as bathroom

NURSING DIAGNOSES	OUTCOME CRITERIA	INTERVENTIONS
	• Describes realistic plan for home maintenance - housekeeping - meal preparation - laundry - child care	• Facilitate identification of others to assist with housekeeping - support persons - religious affiliation - home health/housekeeping • Discuss "essential" versus "nice to do" housework while maintaining bed rest • Discuss, model ways to ask for and accept support
	• Patient/significant other positively acknowledge role changes	• Acknowledge challenge of role changes; provide opportunity to express feelings, concerns, frustrations • Identify potential areas of conflict and plan ways to minimize these areas
		RATIONALE: *Bed rest or severely restricted activities usually accompany home care of PTL. Assisting with plans for managing care of self, family, home, or work is an essential part of discharge planning.*

OTHER LESS COMMON NURSING DIAGNOSES: *Infection; High Risk for Injury (fetus); Altered Tissue Perfusion (placenta); Constipation; Anticipatory Grieving; Diversional Activity Deficit; Noncompliance; Altered Sexuality Patterns; Spiritual Distress; Ineffective Management of Therapeutic Regimen; Impaired Home Maintenance Management*

ESSENTIAL DISCHARGE CRITERIA

- Shows no fetal stress
- Experiences no progression of cervical dilation or UC
- Demonstrates uterine palpation, fetal movement count
- Describes medication routine and strategies to minimize UC
- Possesses follow-up appointments, when to call PCP, emergency phone numbers

RUPTURE OF MEMBRANE (SPONTANEOUS PRETERM)

NURSING DIAGNOSES	OUTCOME CRITERIA	INTERVENTIONS
1 High Risk for Infection *r.t. ruptured amniotic membrane, vaginal tract flora, amniotic fluid bacteria*	• Shows normal VS	• Assess VS q4h; report temperature > 38°C (100.4°F)
	• CBC WNL	• Monitor CBC; note/report elevated WBC count • Administer antibiotics as ordered
	• No malodorous or purulent discharge from vagina; uterus nontender	• Assess vaginal discharge, uterine tenderness and/or irritability q4h • Discuss s/s of amnionitis, vaginitis, importance of reporting to PCP
	• No UC	• Assess for UC • Do not perform vaginal exams, unless by PCP order
	• FHR WNL for gestation • Fetal activity WNL for gestation	• Assess FHR and fetal activity q4-8h, as indicated
		RATIONALE: *SPROM may be precipitated by bacterial invasion of amniotic fluid; or infection may occur retrograde via the cervix into the uterine cavity.*
2 High Risk for Injury (fetus) *r.t. altered umbilical cord blood flow, cord compression, inadequate amniotic fluid*	• Fetus shows movement and FHR WNL for gestation - NST reactive - BPP ≥ 8	• Assess FHR; movement continuously monitored for first 24-48 h, then q4-8h • Assess fetal position using Leopold's movement • Anticipate possible cord prolapse and emergency response based on gestation/family – PCP plan • Follow fetal ultrasound for growth and BPP
		RATIONALE: *Amniotic fluids provide a cushion for fetus and minimize potential of compression, contractures, or lung hypoplasia.*

NURSING DIAGNOSES	OUTCOME CRITERIA	INTERVENTIONS
3 Anxiety *r.t. possible preterm delivery, cesarean birth, unknown fetal outcome*	• Shows decreased anxiety	• Facilitate discussion of fears, concerns • Involve support persons
	• Verbalizes realistic plans for the pregnancy	• Provide tour of NICU as indicated • Discuss potential outcome scenarios given the clinical picture; assist in dealing with ambiguity of outcome expectations • Provide written information regarding PTL, delivery, neonatal problems of current gestation
		RATIONALE: *Information provided to meet the patient's and family's concerns offers a realistic framework for the family to use in coping with SPROM.*
4 Knowledge Deficit *r.t. lack of experience with SPROM*	• Verbalizes s/s of infection	• Discuss s/s to be reported to PCP - change in vaginal discharge - temperature > 38°C (100.4°F) - flu-like feelings - uterine tenderness • Provide printed materials to reinforce teaching • Thoroughly document discharge teaching
	• Verbalizes plan for follow-up	• Stress importance of regular follow-up with PCP
	• Demonstrates fetal movement counts	• Teach fetal movement counts, when to call PCP
		RATIONALE: *Prompt detection of amnionitis/chorioamnionitis is essential to maximize healthy fetal outcomes.*

NURSING DIAGNOSES	OUTCOME CRITERIA	INTERVENTIONS
5 Caregiver Role Strain *r.t. bed rest, young children in home, work restrictions*	• Verbalizes plan for self-care at home	• Discuss strategies for self-care given bed rest limitations - cooler at bedside/couch filled with juices, snacks, sandwich - position phone, radio, TV, reading material within easy reach - if stairs in the home, set up self in area on same floor as bathroom
	• Verbalizes plan for home maintenance - housekeeping - meal preparation - laundry - child care	• Facilitate identification of others to assist with housekeeping - support persons - religious affiliation - home health/housekeeping • Discuss "essential" versus "nice to do" housework while maintaining bed rest • Discuss, model ways to ask for and accept support
	• Patient/significant other positively acknowledge role changes	• Acknowledge challenge of role changes; provide opportunity to express feelings, concerns, frustrations • Identify potential areas of conflict and plan ways to minimize these areas
		RATIONALE: *Bed rest or severely restricted activities usually accompany home care of SPROM. Assisting with plans for the effect on self, family, home, or work is an essential part of discharge planning.*

OTHER LESS COMMON NURSING DIAGNOSES: *Constipation; Anticipatory Grieving; Divisional Activity Deficit; Noncompliance; Altered Sexuality Patterns; Spiritual Distress; Ineffective Management of Therapeutic Regimen; Impaired Home Maintenance Management*

ESSENTIAL DISCHARGE CRITERIA

- Afebrile, uterus nontender, no UC
- FHR, fetal movement WNL
- Demonstrates uterine palpation, fetal movement counts
- Verbalizes medication routine
- Possesses list of follow-up appointments, when to call PCP, emergency phone numbers

ANTEPARTUM

THROMBOEMBOLIC DYSFUNCTION

NURSING DIAGNOSES	OUTCOME CRITERIA	INTERVENTIONS
1 Altered Tissue Perfusion *r.t. deep vein thrombosis, thrombophlebitis*	• Shows no compromise in circulation to extremities (legs) - CRT < 3 sec - extremities warm - palpable pulses	• Assess and monitor circulation to extremities q4h - temperature, color, pulses, CRT, swelling, movement, strength • Elevate legs; provide foot cradle • Minimize external compression - no pillow behind knee - no crossing legs • Maintain complete bed rest during acute phase • Encourage repositioning q2h • Measure and document calf and thigh measurements • Provide antiembolic stockings as ordered • Assess skin integrity
	• Shows no signs of deep vein thrombosis - no chest pain - no cough - no headache - no change in LOC	• Assess for s/s of deep vein thrombosis • Monitor coagulation lab work - PT, PTT 1.5 x normal • Administer anticoagulation therapy as ordered • Teach patient to administer anticoagulation therapy; refer to home health services • Teach s/s of deep vein thrombosis
		RATIONALE: *Circulatory compromise due to venous occlusion needs to be identified early to minimize complications.*
2 Impaired Gas Exchange *r.t. pulmonary deep vein thrombrosis*	• Demonstrates easy respirations - no SOB - no chest pain - no pallor - no anxiety - ABGs WNL	• Assess respirations, breath sounds q4h • Encourage TCDB q2-4h • Avoid exertion; maintain bed rest during acute phase • Monitor blood gas; administer O_2 as ordered • Assess and report signs of pulmonary embolism

NURSING DIAGNOSES	OUTCOME CRITERIA	INTERVENTIONS
	• Performs self-care without SOB	• Discuss plans for self-care, strategies to minimize stress, fatigue • Discuss s/s to report to PCP in timely fashion
		RATIONALE: *Common complication of thrombophlebitis is movement of embolus to lung. Attention to pulmonary assessment is essential.*
3 Caregiver Role Strain *r.t. bed rest, lack of support for self-care, child care, and home maintenance management*	• Describes plan for self-care at home	• Discuss strategies for self-care given bed rest limitations - cooler at bedside/couch filled with juices, snacks, sandwich - position phone, radio, TV, reading material within easy reach - if stairs in the home, set up self-care area on same floor as bathroom
	• Describes realistic plan for home maintenance - housekeeping - meal preparation - laundry - child care	• Facilitate identification of others to assist with housekeeping - support persons - religious affiliation - home health/housekeeping • Discuss "essential" versus "nice to do" housework while maintaining bed rest • Discuss, model ways to ask for and accept support
	• Patient/significant other positively acknowledge role changes	• Acknowledge challenge of role changes; provide opportunity to express feelings, concerns, frustrations • Identify potential areas of conflict and plan ways to minimize these areas
		RATIONALE: *Bed rest or severely restricted activities usually accompany home care. Assisting with plans for managing care of self, family, home, or work is an essential part of discharge planning.*

OTHER LESS COMMON NURSING DIAGNOSES: *Anxiety; Knowledge Deficit; Constipation; Diversional Activity Deficit; Altered Sexuality Patterns; Ineffective Management of Therapeutic Regimen; Impaired Home Maintenance Management*

ESSENTIAL DISCHARGE CRITERIA

- Shows no fetal stress
- Demonstrates medication administration, routine
- Verbalizes s/s of circulatory compromise, when to call PCP
- PT, PTT in therapeutic range for anticoagulation therapy
- Acknowledges plan for follow-up

URINARY TRACT INFECTION

NURSING DIAGNOSES	OUTCOME CRITERIA	INTERVENTIONS

See "Infectious Disorders" care plan in Antepartal Section

NURSING DIAGNOSES	OUTCOME CRITERIA	INTERVENTIONS
1 High Risk for Injury (maternal, fetal) *r.t. toxins secondary to acute genitourinary or other systemic infection*	• Exhibits no s/s of infection - no fever, chills - no pain (flank or lumbar) - no nausea, anorexia, vomiting - no bacteria	• Monitor VS q4h • Assess for complaints of pain, fever, chills
	• Shows FHT WNL - normal fetal activity	• Assess FHT, q4-8h per unit standard
	• Verbalizes knowledge of s/s of infection to report to physician	• Instruct to report fever, chills, and flank pain immediately to physician • Administer prescribed medications; assess effects, side effects • Educate patient regarding correct methods of medication administration at home • Instruct to recognize the s/s of PTL and need to seek immediate medical attention
		RATIONALE: *UTI is a common infection for pregnant women and can lead to PTL and pyelonephritis if not treated promptly.*
2 Pain *r.t. dysuria, flank pain secondary to UTI*	• Drinks ≥ 64 oz per 2000 mL of appropriate fluids q24h	• Instruct to drink a minimum of 8 to 10 glasses of fluids/day and avoid liquids with caffeine, alcohol (should always be avoided in pregnancy), and carbonation
	• Is free of dysuria	• Suggest cranberry juice to help relieve burning, urgency, and frequency
		RATIONALE: *Drinking adequate fluids will help to relieve symptoms of urinary tract discomfort. Alcohol, carbonated beverages, and caffeine should be avoided as they are bladder irritants.*

NURSING DIAGNOSES	OUTCOME CRITERIA	INTERVENTIONS
3 Knowledge Deficit *r.t. lack of information about prevention and treatment of UTI*	• Verbalizes knowledge of methods to prevent UTIs	• Provide information about hygienic measures to prevent UTIs - void before and after intercourse and use lubrication as necessary - wipe from front to back after voiding or defecating and use good handwashing - drink adequate fluids daily (8-10 glasses) - void as frequently as the need arises; avoid prolonged intervals without voiding
	• Agrees to complete treatment and obtain follow-up care	• Instruct to finish medication regime even if symptoms of UTI subside • Encourage to seek follow-up treatment • Teach s/s to report to physician
		RATIONALE: *Using hygienic measures helps to prevent the occurrence of UTI by avoiding the introduction of organisms and preventing their ability to colonize the urinary tract.*
4 Altered Urinary Elimination *r.t. infection*	• Urinary elimination WNL - no urgency or frequency - no dysuria, bladder cramps, or spasms - no itching, warmth during urination - no nocturia - no low back pain - no malaise, nausea, vomiting - no chills or fever	• Assess s/s q2-4h • Assess lab parameters q shift • Provide sitz bath prn
	• Shows no RBC, WBC in urine	• Obtain clean catch urine for urinalysis and culture • Dip urine for presence of RBC, WBC
	• Has bacterial count WNL	• Report results to PCP • Reculture in 1-2 weeks
	• Complies with antibiotic therapy	• Administer medication as ordered

NURSING DIAGNOSES	OUTCOME CRITERIA	INTERVENTIONS
	• Communicates accurate understanding how UTI is contracted and managed and how recurrence can be prevented	• Teach to wipe from front to back, clean with soap and water after BMs, and empty bladder q2-3h

RATIONALE: *Early detection leads to early intervention. Perineal hygiene prevents UTIs while promoting comfort.*

OTHER LESS COMMON NURSING DIAGNOSES:
Anxiety; Nutrition, Less than body requirements

ESSENTIAL DISCHARGE CRITERIA

- FHR WNL
- Denies pain, frequency, dysuria
- Urinalysis and culture WNL
- Has no s/s of infection
- Exhibits no s/s of PTL
- Verbalizes knowledge of treatment and preventative measures specific to invading organism
- Verbalizes knowledge of and agreement to take medications exactly as ordered

INTRAPARTUM

CONTENTS

LABOR ASSESSMENT AND SUPPORT

NURSING DIAGNOSES	OUTCOME CRITERIA	INTERVENTIONS
1 Pain *r.t. uterine contractions, positioning, fear, ineffective coping*	• Follows breathing/relaxation techniques - states pain is decreased - is able to rest or relax in between contractions - labor progress (cervical dilation) is seen	• Assess response to labor - acknowledge the presence of pain - encourage and assist with position of comfort - offer pain relief measures: warm shower or bath, heating pad, cool cloth, back rub, jacuzzi - facilitate/teach breathing/relaxation techniques - explain causes of pain in labor - provide factual information regarding anticipated effects of pain medications - medicate for pain as ordered and at patient's request - assess response to medications and interventions - assess need for regional analgesia (if available) **RATIONALE:** *Unrelieved pain can decrease coping abilities and inhibit the normal progress of labor.*
2 Anxiety *r.t. unknown maternal and neonatal outcomes*	• Mother/partner participates in stress control - verbalize at least one to two concerns of labor/delivery process - state one personal coping mechanism	• Assess level of anxiety: mild, moderate, severe, panic • Provide calm reassurance and comfort - make frequent contact with client and support person(s) or stay with constantly as necessary and available - assess client and support person(s) ability to make decisions and how demands are processed and handled - speak slowly and calmly when communicating with client and support person(s) - convey a sense of calm, confidence, and empathy through touching, allowing effective communication, quiet presence, and praise **RATIONALE:** *Being able to identify anxiety and control it helps to expedite labor/delivery process.*

NURSING DIAGNOSES	OUTCOME CRITERIA	INTERVENTIONS
3 Knowledge Deficit *r.t. unfamiliarity with situation*	• Mother/partner demonstrate correct breathing, relaxation techniques - verbalizes increased comfort through use of breathing techniques and self-comfort measures - partner demonstrates adequate and effective comfort measures	• Facilitate/support partner role in mother's comfort and support • Demonstrate or suggest the following comfort activities: hand-holding, wiping face with cool compresses, offering ice chips, giving back massage, positioning with pillows, assisting with ambulation • Demonstrate or reinforce support person(s) knowledge of relaxation and breathing techniques • Accept and encourage support person's individual style of labor coaching • Offer explanation in meaningful terms of all procedures done to mother
		RATIONALE: *If client and partner are well informed, effective labor progression is facilitated.*
4 Altered Family Processes *r.t. mother's hospitalization and concentration on birthing process*	• Verbalize feelings about hospital situation to nurse or staff members	• Create a private and supportive hospital birth environment for mother and partner • Provide mother/partner with accurate information and answers to questions • Demonstrate active listening to promote communication
	• Participate in labor/birth process as needed	• Involve support person(s) in care of mother
	• Demonstrate mutual support for each other	• Help support person(s) to adapt expectations of mother in a realistic manner
		RATIONALE: *Involvement in labor process facilitates interaction between mother and partner.*

NURSING DIAGNOSES	OUTCOME CRITERIA	INTERVENTIONS
5 High Risk for Fluid Volume Deficit *r.t. decreased oral intake; nausea and vomiting; insensible fluid losses associated with breathing techniques (extreme exercise and diaphoresis)*	• Shows no s/s of fluid deficit - balanced I&O - moist mucous membranes - no heavy bleeding - no signs of fetal stress	• Assess excess fluid loss - pant/blow breathing - vomiting/ nausea - diaphoresis • Record I&O • Monitor for signs of early fetal stress related to maternal dehydration • Offer clear fluids/ice chips/popsicles as tolerated • Administer IV fluids as ordered **RATIONALE:** *Early assessment and intervention minimizes potential for dehydration.*
6 High Risk for Injury (fetus) *r.t. hypoxia* *(Refer to "Fetal Stress" care plan)*	• Experiences prompt detection/management of fetal distress	• Establish baseline FHT and evaluate in relationship to contraction pattern • Initiate EFM as indicated by - FHR > 160 or < 120 - deceleration is auscultated • Continue to assess fetal response to labor using the appropriate method - continuous EFM - intermittent auscultation • Initiate interventions for signs of fetal stress - lateral position - IV fluids - O_2 by face mask @ 8-10 L/min - notify physician or nurse midwife of findings and interventions - anticipate tocolytic **RATIONALE:** *Assessment prompts early detection, management of distress, positioning, hydration, etc., and enhances placental circulation and fetal oxygenation.*

OTHER LESS COMMON NURSING DIAGNOSES: *High Risk for Injury (maternal); Fear; Fatigue; Ineffective Family Coping; Ineffective Individual Coping*

ESSENTIAL DISCHARGE CRITERIA

- Verbalizes adequate pain relief in labor
- Demonstrates effective coping mechanisms during labor process
- Verbalizes and demonstrates breathing techniques and self-directed comfort measures during labor process
- Maintains stable fluid volume status throughout labor

DYSFUNCTIONAL LABOR

NURSING DIAGNOSES	OUTCOME CRITERIA	INTERVENTIONS
1 Knowledge Deficit *r.t. lack of experience of labor, dysfunctional labor*	• Verbalizes understanding of labor process and options available and is able to cooperate in alternative birth plan	• Explain expected treatment and outcomes - answer questions about labor progress - allow patient to express feelings - encourage support person to remain with patient **RATIONALE:** *Increased knowledge related to the labor process helps the mother maintain positive goals and participate in the plan.*
2 Anxiety *r.t. potential Cesarean birth, lack of knowledge regarding labor*	• Maintains a positive attitude and expresses realistic expectations about outcome	• Monitor progress of labor, documenting dilation and pattern - explain process to patient and support person - maintain positive attitude about ability to cope - reassure patient and support person about well-being of fetus **RATIONALE:** *Reducing anxiety reduces stress and increases coping with labor process. Stress can cause vasoconstrictions and decrease placental perfusion.*
3 Pain *r.t. labor, dysfunctional uterine contraction pattern*	• Patient verbalizes increased comfort; shows reduced tension and anxiety with UC	• Use nonpharmacological measures such as position change, low back pressure, and visualization to increase relaxation, breathing techniques • Provide analgesic or anesthesia as appropriate with order • Document response to UC and coping ability **RATIONALE:** *Pain perception may be intensified by tension, fear, or anxiety. Pain causes maternal stress.*

NURSING DIAGNOSES	OUTCOME CRITERIA	INTERVENTIONS
4 High Risk of Infection *r.t. frequent vaginal exams, IUPC*	• Exhibits no signs of infection - afebrile - FHR WNL	• Maintain aseptic technique, minimal vaginal exams, perineal cleanliness • Note characteristics and odor of amniotic fluid • Monitor and document VS and FHR **RATIONALE:** *Invasive procedures increase potential risk of infection, especially with prolonged rupture of membranes.*

OTHER LESS COMMON NURSING DIAGNOSES: *Fluid Volume Deficit; Urinary Retention; High Risk for Injury (to fetus)*

ESSENTIAL DISCHARGE CRITERIA

- Demonstrates positive attitude and realistic expectations about outcome
- Exhibits no signs of infection
- Is involved with alternative birth planning
- Is no longer experiencing abnormal labor pattern

LABOR INDUCTION/AUGMENTATION

NURSING DIAGNOSES	OUTCOME CRITERIA	INTERVENTIONS
1 High Risk for Injury (maternal) *r.t. inability to proceed with labor; uterine rupture, abruptio placentae, water intoxication*	• Shows Bishop score > 7 for primipara, > 5 for multipara	• Perform Bishop score to assess cervical readiness
	• Shows maternal VS WNL	• Monitor maternal VS q30-60 min per institutional standards
	• Shows FHR WNL	• Monitor FHR continuously
	• Maintain contractions regularity in frequency, duration, and intensity	• Monitor, administer ordered oxytocin - start primary infusion line, piggy-back oxytocin - follow orders for oxytocin dosage, administration (not to exceed 20 mU/min at physician's order) • Provide continuous uterine contraction monitoring
	• Shows cervical changes progressing toward complete	• Perform vaginal exam as indicated - graph labor curve • Assess contraction pattern
	• Shows no s/s of hyperstimulation - no contractions > q2 min - no contractions > 90 sec - no resting uterine tone > 20 mmHg - no intrauterine pressure > 90 mmHg	• Assess uterine activity q15 min • Monitor for s/s of hyperstimulation - electronically monitor UC and resting tone - initiate internal uterine pressure catheter monitoring per orders - if hyperstimulation occurs, stop oxytocin, continuing primary IV, call PCP - administer tocolytic agent per orders - keep patient informed of progress • Assess for s/s of uterine rupture, notify PCP immediately, anticipate cesarean delivery
	• Shows no s/s of water intoxication - no headache - no nausea or vomiting - no urinary output - no hypotension - no tachycardia - no arrhythmia - no mental convulsion	• Assess for s/s of water intoxication qh, report to PCP - monitor urine output - assess BP, HR, CNS

NURSING DIAGNOSES	OUTCOME CRITERIA	INTERVENTIONS
		RATIONALE: *Hypertonic uterus increases the risk of uterine rupture and abruptio placentae. Oxytocin increases risk of water intoxication.*
2 High Risk for Injury (fetal) *r.t. hypertonic uterus*	• Maintains FHR WNL - accelerates 6-10 bpm during contractions, maternal activity, or fetal movement	• Provide continuous EFM; assess q15 min for baseline rate, variability, periodic and nonperiodic change, reassuring and nonreassuring characteristics
	• Shows no variable decelerations, persistent bradycardia, sinusoidal FHR pattern	• Identify, report, and manage stressed fetus - place gravida in left-lateral position - stop oxytocin; increase plain IV infusion - administer 0_2 at 8-10 L/min per face mask - suspect fetal hypoxia, acidosis, if persistent bradycardia - report; expect prompt cesarean section
		RATIONALE: *Hypertonic uterus interrupts blood flow to the fetus, increasing the risk of fetal hypoxia.*
3 Pain *r.t. oxytocic effect on uterus*	• Verbalizes understanding of oxytocin therapy: rationale, expected effects • Verbalizes fears, concerns	• Reduce anxiety; establish trust - explain oxytocin therapy, effects, expected course of augmented labor - remind that you will stay with her - include support persons - provide progress reports
	• Reports reasonable comfort between contractions	• Evaluate, manage pain - review/reinforce breathing, relaxation techniques - perform comfort measures: massage, repositioning, diversion - provide ordered analgesics - assist with epidural/intrathecal pain management
		RATIONALE: *Artificial stimulation of labor may be less amenable to nonpharmacologic strategies.*

OTHER LESS COMMON NURSING DIAGNOSES: *Anxiety; Altered Family Processes; Fear; Fluid Volume Excess; Knowledge Deficit; Sleep Pattern Disturbance.*

ESSENTIAL DISCHARGE CRITERIA

- Not applicable

PROLAPSED UMBILICAL CORD

NURSING DIAGNOSES	OUTCOME CRITERIA	INTERVENTIONS
1 High Risk for Injury (fetus) *r.t. interruption of blood flow and 2° prolapsed cord*	• Shows FHR WNL	• Check FHR after ROM • Identify, manage fetal presentation, position, cord prolapse - perform sterile vaginal examination - move presenting part off cord if possible; hold in position until delivery - cover prolapsed cord protruding from vagina with sterile, warm N/S dressing; do not handle or try to reinsert • Monitor, protect safety of fetus - continuously monitor FHR - place gravida in all-fours position - administer ordered IV fluids - administer tocolytic as ordered
	• Delivers viable infant	• Prepare for cesarean delivery - notify neonatal staff of imminent delivery of potentially compromised infant - keep resuscitation equipment available - explain all procedures and ongoing status to mother and family
		RATIONALE: *Prevent further fetal hypoxia, injury, and altered tissue perfusion. Minimize complications and possible fetal death.*
2 Fear *r.t. prolapsed cord, threat to fetal well-being, 2° prolapsed cord*	• Gravida/partner verbalize concerns	• Encourage expressions of feelings, concerns
	• Couple acknowledges information (verbally or nonverbally)	• Inform of potential complications of prolapse - need for immediate cesarean delivery - potentially jeopardized fetus
	• Couple identifies object of fear	• Assist expectant couple to validate source of fear and give support to assist with fear

NURSING DIAGNOSES	OUTCOME CRITERIA	INTERVENTIONS
		RATIONALE: *Prompt nursing and medical attention attempts to minimize fetal damage. Educating and supporting client/family will lower fear that compromises compliance and recovery.*

OTHER LESS COMMON NURSING DIAGNOSES:
High Risk for Infection; Knowledge Deficit; Anxiety; Anticipatory Grieving

ESSENTIAL DISCHARGE CRITERIA

- Not applicable

FETAL STRESS

NURSING DIAGNOSES	OUTCOME CRITERIA	INTERVENTIONS
1 **Impaired Gas Exchange (high risk for)** *r.t. altered placental perfusion, reduction of O_2 levels*	• Shows FHR WNL – 120-160 bpm - short-term variability present - long-term variability normal	• Monitor, manage fetal bradycardia - administer O_2 to mother @ 8-10 L/min by mask - place patient on her side - assess for cord prolapse - notify PCP - perform fetal scalp stimulation - anticipate need for amnio-infusion • Monitor, manage fetal tachycardia - administer O_2 to mother @ 8-10 L/min by mask - place patient on her side - assess maternal temperature; administer antipyretic medications as ordered - increase maternal hydration - notify PCP • Monitor, manage late decelerations - administer O_2 to mother @ 8-10 L/min by mask - place patient on her side - assess maternal BP - if Pitocin is being used stop infusion; open mainline - administer tocolytic as ordered - anticipate need for emergency cesarean delivery - notify PCP • Monitor, manage variable decelerations - administer O_2 to mother at 8-10 L/min by mask - check for umbilical cord prolapse - administer amnio-infusion as ordered - change maternal position to side, Trendelenburg's, or "all fours" - provide nondextrose fluid bolus as ordered - perform scalp stimulation - notify PCP

RATIONALE: *Administering O_2 to the mother increases O_2 supply to the fetus. The left lateral position facilitates uteroplacental perfusion. Trendelenburg's position may alleviate pressure on the umbilical cord, decreasing variable decelerations.*

NURSING DIAGNOSES	OUTCOME CRITERIA	INTERVENTIONS
2 Anxiety *r.t. uncertain health status of fetus*	• Mother and significant other demonstrate decreased anxiety	• Keep patient and significant other apprised of changes in fetal status • Remain calm and carry out procedures in an unhurried manner
	• Freely expresses concerns	• Explain all procedures with rationales • Answer questions honestly
		RATIONALE: *Parents need emotional support, a calm environment, and honest explanations in a time of crisis.*

OTHER LESS COMMON NURSING DIAGNOSES: *Powerlessness; High Risk for Altered Parenting; Knowledge Deficit; Situational Low Self-Esteem*

ESSENTIAL DISCHARGE CRITERIA

- Not applicable

VAGINAL DELIVERY

NURSING DIAGNOSES	OUTCOME CRITERIA	INTERVENTIONS
1 High Risk for Fluid Volume Deficit *r.t. hemoconcentration, hemorrhage* *(Refer to "Postpartum Hemorrhage" care plan)*	• Maintains normal BP, pulse	• Assess cause of fluid/blood loss and intervene appropriately to prevent further blood loss • Monitor VS q15 min if evidence of fluid volume deficit is present • Initiate IV therapy for replacement of fluids or blood products and administration of medications as ordered
	• Maintains normal mental status	• Monitor restlessness, confusion
	• Shows blood loss < 500 mL	• Estimate blood loss, weigh pads and linens as indicated
		RATIONALE: *There is a reduction in vascular volume during labor and delivery. This is due to erythropoiesis, muscular activity, and dehydration, which results in hemoconcentration.*
2 Pain *r.t. physical discomfort of the labor and delivery process*	• Verbalizes increased comfort	• Assess physiologic, behavioral, and emotional pain responses • Collaborate with physician regarding pain relief (narcotics, local, pudendal block, epidural, intrathecal anesthesia)
	• Utilizes nonpharmacologic measures to improve comfort	• Facilitate the use of nonpharmacologic pain relief measures (i.e., positioning, effleurage, imagery, focal point, cold/moist compress, therapeutic touch, breathing techniques for pushing)
		RATIONALE: *The pain experienced during delivery is subjective and personal. Nonpharmacologic measures are often effective in relieving stress and reducing pain.*

OTHER LESS COMMON NURSING DIAGNOSES: *Fatigue; Altered Role Performance; High Risk for Activity*

ESSENTIAL DISCHARGE CRITERIA

- Is ready for recovery care
  - VS WNL
  - Lochia WNL

VAGINAL RECOVERY

NURSING DIAGNOSES	OUTCOME CRITERIA	INTERVENTIONS
1 High Risk for Fluid Volume Deficit *r.t. active fluid loss*	• Maintains normal BP and pulse for patient • Maintains balanced I&O	• Monitor VS q15 min x 4, q30min x 2, or per institutional standards • Encourage oral fluids • Initiate IV therapy for administration of fluids, medications, or blood products as ordered • Measure, estimate voiding
	• Displays normal mental status	• Monitor for signs of restlessness, confusion
	• Maintains normal amount of vaginal lochia - < 500 mL blood loss	• Assess every 15 min for - location and tone of fundus - amount of lochia - color of lochia - consistency of lochia - bladder distension - vulvar or vaginal hematomas • Massage uterus q15 min - observe for clots per vagina
		RATIONALE: *Hemoconcentration during labor, due to decreased fluid intake, paired with delivery blood loss places woman at risk.*
2 Fatigue *r.t. increased metabolic demand*	• Identifies measures that will conserve energy	• Provide a quiet, warm, nurturing environment • Promote comfort in supporting tired muscles with pillow and blanket, e.g., position mother on side with pillow behind back for breastfeeding infant • Assist in managing visitors - encourage short periods of visiting • Involve significant others in discussion regarding - support people that can assist the patient with infant care and household chores - instruct patient to rest whenever the infant is asleep

NURSING DIAGNOSES	OUTCOME CRITERIA	INTERVENTIONS
		RATIONALE: *Delivery physically exhausts most women. Physical and psychological restoration must occur for a woman to fully care for herself and her infant.*

OTHER LESS COMMON NURSING DIAGNOSES: *High Risk for Activity Intolerance; Altered Role Performance; Altered Urinary Elimination*

ESSENTIAL DISCHARGE CRITERIA

- Shows VS WNL
- Fundus firm, lochia WNL
- Urinary output WNL
- Identifies measures to reduce energy expenditure
- Verbalizes plan for routine postpartum follow-up

CESAREAN DELIVERY (PRE-OP)

NURSING DIAGNOSES	OUTCOME CRITERIA	INTERVENTIONS
1 Anxiety *r.t. unexpected need for cesarean delivery*	• Patient/family verbalize understanding of need for cesarean delivery; expressing fears and concerns for mother and fetus	• Stay with patient as much as possible - provide emotional support, encouragement - encourage patient/family to express feelings - answer questions calmly - discuss pre-op and procedures, tests, and preparations - discuss post-op course as much as possible **RATIONALE:** *Anxiety decreases when open lines of communication, support, and information are provided.*
2 Knowledge Deficit *r.t. surgical delivery*	• Patient/family verbalize understanding of the cesarean delivery process; express concerns and questions about the cesarean delivery, pre-op and post-op course	• Assess knowledge level and support needs - explain procedures - answer questions about course of cesarean delivery - provide information about what can be expected during and after delivery including routine care of the neonate - provide information about the role a support person plays in the OR - explain procedures, tests planned for the post-op course **RATIONALE:** *Increased knowledge offers patient and family a feeling of more predictability and control in a stressful situation and decreases anxiety.*

OTHER LESS COMMON NURSING DIAGNOSES: *Anticipatory Grieving; Decisional Conflict; Altered Family Process; Fatigue; Ineffective Individual Coping; Powerlessness; Pain*

ESSENTIAL DISCHARGE CRITERIA

- Not applicable

POSTPARTUM

CONTENTS

BREASTFEEDING

NURSING DIAGNOSES	OUTCOME CRITERIA	INTERVENTIONS
1 Ineffective Breastfeeding *r.t. knowledge deficit, mother unable to position infant at breast to promote a successful latch-on response, previous history of breastfeeding failure, interrupted breastfeeding*	• Demonstrates correct positioning of infant for successful latch-on	• Observe mother with infant every feeding, assess using LATCH score • Explain and demonstrate effective infant positioning to promote successful latch-on response • Allow uninterrupted breastfeeding periods
	• Verbalizes correct knowledge about breastfeeding techniques and physiology of breastfeeding	• Reassure mother that she can breastfeed • Provide information on the physiology and psychology of breastfeeding, advantages, techniques, and support sources
	• Mother/family verbalize increased satisfaction with the process by discharge	• Assess support person's knowledge base about breastfeeding, providing education as needed • Discourage use of supplemental feedings/rubber nipples • Refer to lactation consultant as indicated
		RATIONALE: *Information, reinforcement, and support are essential to the success of breastfeeding.*
2 Effective Breastfeeding *r.t. basic knowledge base, maternal confidence*	• Verbalizes satisfaction with the breastfeeding process	• Initiate breastfeeding within the 30-60 min after birth • Assess, reinforce, and add to patient's knowledge base • Demonstrate how to support and position baby and observe LATCH • Discourage use of supplemental bottle feedings/rubber nipples until breastfeeding is well established • Provide anticipatory guidance for infant growth, relief bottles, soothing fussy baby • Provide anticipatory guidance re: partner, returning to work, and other issues facing the breastfeeding family

NURSING DIAGNOSES	OUTCOME CRITERIA	INTERVENTIONS
		RATIONALE: *Positive support and anticipatory guidance promote maintenance of effective breastfeeding.*
3 Interrupted Breastfeeding *r.t. infant illness*	• Maintains milk supply	• Assess previous experience with breastfeeding, breast pumping • Review with mother - techniques to pump breasts manually or with an electric pump - pumping frequency - storage and transport of pumped milk - fluid and nutritional needs • Provide information about electric pump rental
	• Resumes breastfeeding as soon as infant is physiologically able	• Educate and support mother in breastfeeding techniques for the sick/recovering neonate • Provide/facilitate opportunities for neonate to breastfeed - ensure privacy - minimize potential for cold stress, environmental stress - supplement feeding per physician's order • Provide written materials and community resources, i.e., La Leche League, Breastfeeding Consultants
		RATIONALE: *Mothers may provide breast milk for their infants. Mothers who are educated and supported in the breastfeeding process are more likely to be successful.*

OTHER LESS COMMON NURSING DIAGNOSES:
Pain; High Risk for Infection; High Risk for Injury (breast)

ESSENTIAL DISCHARGE CRITERIA

- Demonstrates correct positioning of infant for successful latch-on
- Infant demonstrates regular and sustained suckling at the breast
- Infant has 6-10 wet diapers a day
- Infant has not lost > 10% of birth weight
- Possesses phone numbers of breastfeeding resources

CESAREAN DELIVERY (POST-OP)

NURSING DIAGNOSES	OUTCOME CRITERIA	INTERVENTIONS
1 Pain *r.t. cesarean delivery*	• Affirms pain relief from comfort measures - reports sustained comfort - has relaxed body posture, facial expression	• Assess level of comfort q1-4h - effectiveness of comfort measures q2-4h - use pain scale (0 = no pain to 10 = worst pain) • Provide comfort measures - reposition q1-2h - provide quiet, restful environment - administer pain meds as indicated
		RATIONALE: *Pain relief fosters mobility, which assists the healing process.*
2 High Risk for Infection *r.t. interrupted skin integrity, surgical intervention*	• Exhibits no s/s of infection - VS WNL - clean, intact incision; no drainage	• Monitor for s/s of infection - assess VS per unit standard - inspect sites of potential infection (incision, IV, uterus, bladder-catheter, lungs)
	• Demonstrates effective TCDB	• Encourage TCDB q2h - reinforce use of incentive spirometer
	• Lungs are clear on auscultation	• Assess breath sounds q4h • Teach measures to facilitate effective breathing pattern (splinting, C/DB positioning, position changes) • Administer antibiotics as ordered
		RATIONALE: *Early detection of infection fosters prompt intervention. preventative measures can minimize risk of infection.*

NURSING DIAGNOSES	OUTCOME CRITERIA	INTERVENTIONS
3 Altered Urinary Elimination *r.t. tissue trauma, anesthesia*	• Achieves, maintains normal elimination - balanced I&O - urinary output > 30 mL/h through indwelling catheter - at least one normal bowel movement prior to discharge - ambulates per prescribed routine	• Monitor I&O • Monitor urinary elimination q4h - catheterize prn - assist to stand or to bathroom to void unless contraindicated • Monitor frequency, amount, characteristics of bowel elimination q8h • Provide, encourage high fluid intake • Dangle at 12 h, ambulate by 24 h, and encourage activity as tolerated • Administer stool softeners, enema per orders
		RATIONALE: *Ambulation and high fluid intake foster excretion of anesthetic effects.*
4 Constipation *r.t. decreased mobility, abdominal surgery*	• Affirms knowledge of post-op constipation management	• Discuss diet, fluid, and stool softener regime for post-op home care
		RATIONALE: *Activity fosters return of normal physiologic functions, i.e., peristalsis, urination. Stool softeners ameliorate the effects of post-op constipation.*
5 Knowledge Deficit *r.t. post-op care at home*	• Mother/partner read post-op instructions; ask questions for clarification	• Provide written post-op instructions; review with patient/partner
	• Mother/partner discuss reportable s/s	• Describe, provide list of reportable s/s consistent with type of surgery
	• Mother/partner describe activity limitations and length, diet modifications, medications, follow-up schedule	• Explain home care requirements; verify written follow-up appointments
		RATIONALE: *A knowledgeable, competent patient is likely to manage her own post-op recovery at home with a minimum of untreated adverse trends.*

OTHER LESS COMMON NURSING DIAGNOSES: *Fluid Volume Deficit; Altered Nutrition: Less than body requirements; Impaired Skin Integrity; Situational Low Self-Esteem*

ESSENTIAL DISCHARGE CRITERIA

- Shows no s/s of infection
- Maintains normal elimination
- Maintains pain control with comfort measures
- Accurately describes recommended home care, medications, activity, diet, and follow-up

EARLY DISCHARGE (VAGINAL DELIVERY)

NURSING DIAGNOSES	OUTCOME CRITERIA	INTERVENTIONS
1 High Risk for Injury *r.t. childbirth, altered involution*	• Shows VS WNL for postpartal period - BP above 90/60 - temperature < 38°C (100.4°F) - pulse 60-100 bpm • Uterus is firm below umbilicus - lochia will be rubra or serosa, WNL • Perineum is intact or episiotomy approximated without bleeding	• Assess VS • Postpartum physical assessment including breast, nipples, fundus, perineum • Teach and demonstrate application of topical medications • Teach perineal care • Teach use of portable sitz bath bid and prn
		RATIONALE: *Assure early recognition of altered postpartum course.*
2 Pain *r.t. episiotomy, involution, fatigued muscles*	• Verbalizes pain relief • Shows relaxed facial expression	• Assess client's pain using pain scale • Provide comfort measures and analgesic medications as ordered • Discuss nonpharmacologic comfort measures - relaxation breathing - sitz bath - ice • Monitor relief • Provide prescription for home use if ordered
		RATIONALE: *Enhance client comfort.*
3 High Risk for Injury *r.t. altered elimination*	• Shows normal elimination pattern - voids > 200 mL per void	• Assess voiding pattern • Encourage early ambulation • Assess bladder distention and uterine displacement
	• Reports hemorrhoids to be nonpainful	• Assess presence/ status of hemorrhoids • Encourage fluids and fiber in the diet • Administer stool softeners, hemorrhoid preparation as ordered

NURSING DIAGNOSES	OUTCOME CRITERIA	INTERVENTIONS
		RATIONALE: *Client may experience both urine and bowel elimination problems as a result of childbirth process. These include urinary retention and burning as well as constipation and hemorrhoids.*
4 Knowledge Deficit *r.t. continuing needs of self, family, and infant during postpartum period, lack of experience*	• Provides care for self, infant in the hospital	• Keep infant with mother as much as hospital routines allow • Provide written information on self and baby care including warning signs for self and infant - temperature - elimination - nutrition - rest/sleep patterns • Encourage patient to perform as much infant care as possible while in hospital • Encourage questions; provide hospital and physician's phone numbers upon discharge • Plan for physician follow-up for mother or mother and infant • Provide numbers of available parent support groups and/or breastfeeding groups • Schedule home visits as agency policy permits
	• Identifies resources for where to turn for help at home	• Discuss with mother plans for home care, availability of support and resources
	• Demonstrates positive interactions with infant and family	• Observe and record bonding between infant and family • Observe and assess maternal caretaking of infant, feeding, changing diapers, etc.
		RATIONALE: *Assess current caretaking abilities and knowledge base and provide resources for further information.*

OTHER LESS COMMON NURSING DIAGNOSES: *Altered Nutrition: Less than body requirements; Sleep Pattern Disturbance; Altered Health Maintenance; Anxiety; Ineffective Breastfeeding; Fatigue; High Risk for Altered Parenting*

ESSENTIAL DISCHARGE CRITERIA

Maternal

- Is able to move about freely
- Ordered laboratory and x-ray tests are completed
- Arrangements for RhoGAM injection (if applicable) are made
- Uterus is nontender, firm, and below the umbilicus; voiding is normal, emotional well-being is satisfactory

Infant

- VS, especially temperature, WNL
- Displays good suck/swallow reflexes and breathing coordination during feedings
- Shows no Rh or ABO incompatibilities
- Has passed stool and urine
- Arrangements have been made for follow-up lab work and healthcare

GRIEF, PERINATAL LOSS

NURSING DIAGNOSES	OUTCOME CRITERIA	INTERVENTIONS
1 Dysfunctional Grieving *r.t. perinatal loss, 2° to spontaneous abortion, ectopic pregnancy, gestational trophoblastic disease, pre-term delivery, intrauterine fetal death, or neonatal death*	• Verbalizes and demonstrates normal, progressive grieving behaviors	• Assess previous losses, expectations for this pregnancy, coping practices, and sociocultural values and practices • Acknowledge reality of feelings and accept expressions of grief • Use therapeutic communication to encourage verbalizations of feelings and thoughts • Avoid nontherapeutic blockers that minimize feelings and the loss, such as "Don't worry," or "You can have other babies" • Give factual, complete information; repeat clarification as needed (refer to ND #3 Knowledge Deficit) • Provide reassurance of normalcy of feelings and behavior • Maintain confidentiality and provide privacy • Provide consistent caretaker, be available for listening • Prepare for contact with baby if desired (refer to ND #3 Knowledge Deficit) - prepare baby for viewing: groom, dress, and wrap - allow mother to hold baby - provide privacy - offer factual information as well as point out positive characteristics of baby - take pictures, keep on file if parents don't want • Engage support system: family (refer to ND #2 Altered Family Processes), bereavement team, clergy, social worker, support groups, postdischarge resources • Offer sensitive, personalized care for mother including comfort measures, rest, and nutrition • Discuss need to establish own pace of grief resolution and to remove any preparations for newborn at home when ready

NURSING DIAGNOSES	OUTCOME CRITERIA	INTERVENTIONS
		• Discuss use of family planning until full physical and psychological recovery • Document grief support and response on bereavement checklist for continuity of care • Develop method for staff to identify grieving patient to avoid uninformed, insensitive comments
		RATIONALE: *Grief is the expected response after a loss and the process must occur for resolution. Manifestations of grief are individual. Communication facilitates resolution.*
2 Altered Family Processes *r.t. crisis associated with perinatal loss*	• Individual family members express feelings regarding loss	• Discuss that individual family members may not progress toward resolution at the same pace • Provide opportunity to express feelings
	• Family demonstrates mutual support as members progress through grief	• Assess family communication patterns, response to loss, and previous coping practices • Assess family role expectations and sociocultural values and practices • Facilitate verbalization of feelings and thoughts among family members, including children • Provide private time for family members to interact with/without baby • Discuss explanations and announcements to be given to others
		RATIONALE: *All family members experience loss and grieve individually. Children may misunderstand and feel guilty. Communication will facilitate emotional support.*

NURSING DIAGNOSES	OUTCOME CRITERIA	INTERVENTIONS
3 Knowledge Deficit *r.t. options in perinatal loss, lack of familiarity with situation*	• Asks appropriate questions; verbalizes understanding	• Assess knowledge level and readiness to learn • Individualize the pace of information offered and repeat as necessary • Provide verbal information about the grief process and typical feelings to expect • Augment teaching with written information, additional resources available postdischarge, and a postdischarge phone number for contact
	• Makes choices among options	• Provide information for decision-making about mother/baby - birth room assignment - analgesia/anesthesia - support person(s) - contact with baby (what to expect, describe appearance, holding) - photographs, mementos (footprints, identification bracelet, cap, lock of hair, measurements, certificate of birth/death), naming, baptism, autopsy, burial, funeral • Allow time for decision-making • Consult pastoral care and/or social work
		RATIONALE: *Family may need help identifying what needs to be done. Knowledge enhances decision-making, mutual care planning, sense of control, and coping.*
4 Self-Esteem Disturbance *r.t. perceived inadequacy in "normal" reproductive role*	• Expresses feelings of positive self-regard; discusses causes of perinatal loss	• Accept expression of patient's feelings regarding self - reinforce positive expressions of abilities • Assess self-esteem • Assess role expectations • Encourage involvement in decisions about care (refer to ND #3 Knowledge Deficit)

NURSING DIAGNOSES	OUTCOME CRITERIA	INTERVENTIONS
		• Assess family support (refer to ND #3 Knowledge Deficit and ND #2 Altered Family Processes) • Discuss physical changes of involution in a positive manner
		RATIONALE: *Pregnancy loss is often associated with feelings of guilt and inadequacy. Positive reinforcement of abilities and participation in decision-making foster self-esteem.*

OTHER LESS COMMON NURSING DIAGNOSES: *Altered Parenting; Spiritual Distress; Self-Esteem Disturbance; Chronic Low Self-Esteem*

ESSENTIAL DISCHARGE CRITERIA

- Verbalizes feelings of loss
- Discusses grieving as a process to resolve
- Referrals to community support/agencies discussed

POSTPARTUM HEMORRHAGE

NURSING DIAGNOSES	OUTCOME CRITERIA	INTERVENTIONS
1 Fluid Volume Deficit *r.t. hemorrhage*	• Has normal circulating volume - no pallor or cyanosis - normal VS, BP - CRT < 3 sec - normal lochia	• Assess and support circulating volume - administer IV fluids - administer oxytoxic as ordered
	• Shows normal Hb, Hct, clotting factors for postpartal client	• Monitor lab values, report to PCP as indicated • Initiate emergency hemorrhage measures per institutional standards • Administer blood products as ordered • Anticipate need for surgical intervention
		RATIONALE: *These interventions help prevent further blood loss and minimize complications.*
2 High Risk for Activity Intolerance *r.t. deconditioned status, circulatory problems*	• Cares for self and infant	• Assess ADL: advance activity as tolerated • Encourage use of dietary iron supplements • Teach strategies for energy restoration • Assist in identification of in-home support for home maintenance
		RATIONALE: *These measures offer the patient realistic expectations for self-care and minimize postpartal stress.*

OTHER LESS COMMON NURSING DIAGNOSES:
Altered Urinary Elimination; Pain; Impaired Gas Exchange

ESSENTIAL DISCHARGE CRITERIA

- Exhibits no pallor or cyanosis
- Has normal Hb, Hct and clotting factors
- Lochia WNL
- Cares for self and infant

THROMBOPHLEBITIS

NURSING DIAGNOSES	OUTCOME CRITERIA	INTERVENTIONS
1 High Risk for Injury (internal) *r.t. obstructed venous return, embolus*	• Exhibits adequate peripheral blood flow - palpable peripheral pulses - decreasing or no edema - decreasing or no "hot spots"	• Assess and monitor peripheral circulation - check peripheral pulses, edema, CRT, color, and temperature of extremity in area around clot - note edema of lower extremity, increased circumference of extremity compared with unaffected leg at several levels, palpable hard cordlike vein, fever - assist as indicated and monitor results of diagnostic tests such as venogram and Doppler ultrasound • Elevate legs • After acute phase, begin progressive ambulation; provide properly fitting elastic stockings prior to ambulation
	• Shows no s/s of peripheral venous embolism - no apprehension, fear - no chest pain - no dyspnea, cough - no tachycardia - no diaphoresis - no neck vein engorgement	• Monitor q1-2h for mobilization of peripheral venous embolus; note and immediately report s/s of pulmonary embolus - sudden severe chest pain, - increased cough and dyspnea, tachypnea - apprehension and sense of catastrophe - tachycardia, diaphoresis, neck vein engorgement • Initiate emergency treatment
	• Shows PT/PTT lengthened and within therapeutic range	• Administer anticoagulant medication as ordered • Monitor response to anticoagulant therapy - monitor PT and PTT - therapeutically lengthened PT and PTT $1\frac{1}{2}$ to $2 \times$ normal (90-100 sec) - assess and monitor signs of bleeding from puncture sites, gingival oozing; test stool and nasogastric drainage for blood

NURSING DIAGNOSES	OUTCOME CRITERIA	INTERVENTIONS
		RATIONALE: *Early detection permits prompt treatment. Bed rest decreases probability clot will dislodge. Elevation lowers edema and prevents venous stasis. Anticoagulants prevent further clotting. Pulmonary embolism is a major complication of thrombophlebitis.*
2 Pain *r.t. inflammation, edema, venous stasis, and tissue hypoxia*	• Verbalizes pain relief; is able to sleep and rest	• Assess and monitor pain in affected extremity - note tenderness or painful swollen area, sensation of tingling or numbness, leg cramping - note if pain increases in dependent position - assess presence of pain when foot dorsiflexed (Homan's sign) • Administer analgesics as ordered • Position to maximize comfort and safety - change position frequently if mobility is limited - avoid dependent positioning of affected leg or maintain limb in elevated position • Encourage relaxation techniques and provide comfort measures • Encourage questions and verbalization of anxiety and fears
		RATIONALE: *Analgesics will relieve pain. Elevation promotes venous return and helps decrease edema. Other comfort measures promote rest.*
3 Altered Role Performance *r.t. inability to perform role (new parent/mother) as anticipated; decreased maternal/infant interaction*	• Acknowledges impact of situation/condition on maternal role attainment	• Provide frequent contact between mother and infant • Encourage rooming in; keep crib close to mother's bed • Check frequently to help mother with infant

NURSING DIAGNOSES	OUTCOME CRITERIA	INTERVENTIONS
	• Demonstrates ability to function within limitations • Demonstrates bonds of attachment to infant (affectionate behavior toward infant; eager to care for and feed infant; verbalizes positive feelings about infant)	• Encourage and support care and feeding of infant as condition allows
		RATIONALE: *Frequent contact and caring for infant allow patient to function as a mother assisting her with role attainment/performance as expected.*
4 Knowledge Deficit *r.t. disease process, treatment and diagnostic procedures*	• Verbalizes knowledge of self-care strategies • Understanding of disease process and necessary treatment • Able to correctly answer questions about disease and treatment	• Assess knowledge deficit and instruct patient/family about self-care - information concerning the complication and treatment - adequate fluid intake - medications - avoid rubbing or massaging affected area - preventing constipation and avoiding straining with stool - discharge plan, warning signs, and follow-up care - risk factors and possible risk/lifestyle modification - ways to avoid circulatory stasis, e.g., avoid long periods of standing and sitting; avoid crossing legs
		RATIONALE: *Identify and provide early intervention if embolism occurs. Prevent additional complications of mobility.*

OTHER LESS COMMON NURSING DIAGNOSES: *Anxiety; Altered Tissue Perfusion; High Risk for Altered Parenting; High Risk for Altered Family Processes*

ESSENTIAL DISCHARGE CRITERIA

- Displays adequate circulation to extremities: color, pulses, skin temperature WNL
- Verbalizes comfort; absence of acute distress, mental or physical
- Parents demonstrate readiness to assume parenting role and the ability to perform infant care tasks or have assistance
- Verbalizes and demonstrates confidence in ability to manage self-care or has assistance to do so
  - accurately describes activity, dietary and medication regimen
  - identifies s/s requiring medical attention
  - accurately describes plan for follow-up care

TUBERCULOSIS

NURSING DIAGNOSES	OUTCOME CRITERIA	INTERVENTIONS

See "Infectious Disorders" care plan in Antepartal Section

NURSING DIAGNOSES	OUTCOME CRITERIA	INTERVENTIONS
1 Knowledge Deficit *r.t. tuberculosis – spread and treatment*	• Identifies need to learn about tuberculosis	• Teach the patient s/s of tuberculosis: weakness, fatigue, cough, hemoptysis, unexplained weight loss, fever, and night sweats
	• Verbalizes understanding of how tuberculosis is contracted, managed, recurrence prevented	• Explain respiratory and universal precautions to prevent spreading the disease • Teach to cough and sneeze into tissues and dispose in paper bag that will be burned • Instruct the patient and her family concerning s/s of recurring and/or extrapulmonary disease • Teach importance of keeping follow-up appointments and compliance with therapy regimen
		RATIONALE: *Decrease the spread of disease.*
2 Altered Parenting *r.t. infection*	• Continues breastfeeding and providing infant care	• Encourage breastfeeding
		RATIONALE: *Small concentrations of antitubercular drugs in breast milk do not produce toxicity. Facilitate attachment through positive planning activities.*
3 Fear *r.t. chronic communicable disease*	• Verbalizes fear of separation	• Discuss isolation plan • Discuss plan for contact with infant, providing care
		RATIONALE: *Separation of the infant from the mother is necessary only if she has active disease pending treatment, requires prolonged hospitalization, or is noncompliant with treatment.*

NURSING DIAGNOSES	OUTCOME CRITERIA	INTERVENTIONS
4 **Ineffective Airway Clearance** *r.t. pulmonary secretions*	• Exhibits no s/s of hypoxia - no SOB - no cyanosis, pallor - RR WNL	• Teach coughing and deep breathing exercises • Monitor respiratory status/TPR • Auscultate breath sounds frequently
	• Can list drugs, dose, actions, and side effects of prescribed medications	• Administer ordered antibiotics and antitubercular agents with food • Watch for and teach side effects of drugs • Isolate infectious patient in a negative pressure room • Provide for plenty of rest
		RATIONALE: *Pulmonary secretions need to be cleared from the airway to allow adequate ventilation.*
5 **Altered Nutrition: Less than body requirements** *r.t. changes in metabolism*	• Explains how a nutritionally adequate diet will be achieved	• Provide well-balanced, high protein, high caloric foods, frequently, in small amounts • Monitor weight
		RATIONALE: *Provide nutrients for healing and support fetal growth.*

OTHER LESS COMMON NURSING DIAGNOSES: *Impaired Gas Exchange; Anxiety; Ineffective Coping Patterns*

ESSENTIAL DISCHARGE CRITERIA

- No s/s of disease
- Sputum negative
- Verbalizes plans for compliance with drug therapy regimen

VAGINAL DELIVERY (POSTPARTUM)

NURSING DIAGNOSES	OUTCOME CRITERIA	INTERVENTIONS
1 Pain *r.t. laceration, episiotomy, hemorrhoids, swelling, bruising or hematoma; uterine cramping*	• Verbalizes increased comfort	• Teach comfort measures - ice pack - heat lamp - anesthetic cream or spray - sitz bath (warm or cool) - witch hazel pads • Inspect perineum; explain cause of pain and how long it will last • Explore various methods of pain relief (relaxation, ambulation, position, diet) • Administer analgesic medication as ordered • K-pad to abdomen for cramping • Back rub (for lower back) • Positioning • Time analgesics 20-30 min before breastfeeding **RATIONALE:** *Promote comfort, decrease swelling, and promote healing.*
2 High Risk for Fluid Volume Deficit *r.t. hemorrhage secondary to uterine atony, retained placental fragments, cervical lacerations* *(Refer to "Postpartum Hemorrhage" care plan)*	• VS stable and WNL • Shows lochia WNL • Fundus is firm	• Assess VS per unit standard • Monitor amount and character of lochia - first hour q15 min - second hour q30 min - first 24 h q4h • If heavy, reassess source of bleeding, uterine tone, and degree of bladder distension • Gently massage fundus • Expel clots • Teach expected regression during involution and need to report clots and increased lochia **RATIONALE:** *Prevent possible fluid volume deficit. Prevent hemorrhage by maintaining muscle tone.*

NURSING DIAGNOSES	OUTCOME CRITERIA	INTERVENTIONS
3 Altered Urinary Elimination *r.t. perineal edema, anesthesia, trauma*	• Resumes normal pattern of urinary elimination as indicated by voiding q4-8h post delivery • Nondistended bladder voiding is increased 200 mL in first two voids and no discomfort with voiding	• Ensure adequate fluid intake • Check bladder for distention • Encourage early voiding and ambulation • Catheterize prior to overdistention if indicated • Monitor voiding patterns and amounts • Assist with voiding by running water, peri-care, warm sitz bath
		RATIONALE: *Prevent urinary retention. Ensure bladder functioning and adequacy of emptying.*
4 High Risk for Impaired Skin Integrity *r.t. breastfeeding*	• Meets goals of lactation or suppression with minimal discomfort	• Lactation - inspect nipples for redness, fissures or blisters - observe feeding position - check latching on and tongue lip placement - teaching alternate breastfeeding positions to decrease trauma - teach breast hygiene, keep clean, well-fitting bra (unlined), cotton breast pads - teach detachment techniques - offer mild analgesic 30 min prior to feeding
		RATIONALE: *Decrease potential for loss of skin integrity due to ineffective breastfeeding techniques.*

NURSING DIAGNOSES	OUTCOME CRITERIA	INTERVENTIONS
5 High Risk for Alteration in Parenting *r.t. failure to take on role of mother*	• Provides infant care and verbalizes awareness of infant cues (i.e., hunger, sleep, stimulation)	• Teach physical caretaking skills (diapering, bathing) • Facilitate participation in infant's care • Have infant remain in room with mother if conditions permit • Provide infant care if mother too exhausted to participate • Refer for community health follow-up if mother at risk for failure to assume maternal role • Encourage nurturing of infant and bonding
		RATIONALE: *Provide opportunity for assuming new role as mother with support and encouragement.*

OTHER LESS COMMON NURSING DIAGNOSES: *Constipation; Impaired Skin Integrity; High Risk for Infection; Ineffective Individual Coping*

ESSENTIAL DISCHARGE CRITERIA

- Able to employ measures to increase comfort level
- Lochia remains WNL
- Resumes normal elimination pattern
- Establishes feeding method of choice with minimal discomfort
- Demonstrates competence in infant caregiving activities

NEWBORN

NEWBORN

CONTENTS

CIRCUMCISION

NURSING DIAGNOSES	OUTCOME CRITERIA	INTERVENTIONS
1 **High Risk for Infection** *r.t. invasive procedure of circumcision*	• Is free of signs of infection at circumcision site	• Wash hands and teach parents to do so before caring for circumcision site • Assess circumcision site for cleanliness and healing - no swelling - no redness - no purulent drainage • With each diaper change, cleanse penis with clear, warm water gently squeezed from a cotton ball • With each diaper change, following cleansing, apply petrolatum gauze loosely over penis to reduce bleeding and encrustation; if plastibell used, do not use dressing or petroleum jelly • Monitor axillary temperature q4h
	• Parents discuss/demonstrate correct circumcision care - reiterate s/s of infection - ask appropriate questions - perform return demonstration	• Explain and demonstrate how to reduce risk of infection • Review s/s of infection
		RATIONALE: *Complete healing of circumcision does not occur until 7-10 days after procedure. Careful cleansing reduces risk of contamination from fecal matter. Petrolatum gauze serves as a protective layer against abrasion from diaper. Abrasion could lead to infection.*

NURSING DIAGNOSES	OUTCOME CRITERIA	INTERVENTIONS
2 Pain *r.t. irritation of the denuded glans and trauma of surgical incision*	• Pain is minimized	• Provide comfort measures to neonate during surgical procedure such as - talking softly - gently holding of his head - offering a pacifier • Encourage mother to hold, rock, and cuddle neonate after procedure • Perform comfort measures - apply diapers loosely and change frequently after each voiding or BM - generously apply petrolatum gauze around circumcision site for 24 h and replace dressing with each diaper change - place newborn in side-lying position with needed linen supports and diaper off - continue to assess neonate for reactions to pain after procedure, such as crying, total body movements, change in eating patterns, change in sleeping patterns, change in urinary patterns
	• Parents perform comfort measures	• Demonstrate how to hold, rock, and cuddle neonate • Explain s/s of pain • Reinforce need to report to PCP if neonate is inconsolable
		RATIONALE: *Reaction to pain may be subdued when caregiver or parent provides distraction. Petrolatum dressings protect incision from contact with urine and prevent diaper from sticking to circumcision site. Despite controversy over how mature a newborn's neurologic system is, pain perception seems to exist based on reaction to painful stimuli.*

NURSING DIAGNOSES	OUTCOME CRITERIA	INTERVENTIONS
3 Knowledge Deficit *r.t. care for circumcision and prevention of complications*	• Parents express and demonstrate ability to care for circumcision and prevent complications	• Develop individualized teaching plan based on assessment of knowledge • Provide information, demonstrations, practice opportunities, and other teaching modalities as appropriate - gently cleanse circumcision site with warm water to remove feces and urine, wiping away from site - apply petrolatum and dressing as needed after each diaper change, unless plastibell is used - apply diaper lightly after each voiding - if dressing becomes stuck or dry, moisten with warm water before attempting removal - demonstrate application of appropriate amount of manual pressure for 5-10 min, should active bleeding be observed • Teach parents to be aware of s/s, behaviors indicating complications of infection, hemorrhage, urinary retention, or altered tissue perfusion - be aware that a foul-smelling, purulent exudate is abnormal and report to healthcare provider - report any frank bleeding or continuous oozing to healthcare provider - report any blue or black discoloring of circumcision site immediately - diapers should be sufficiently wet after each feeding - report failure of circumcision to heal completely in 7-10 days, regardless of method used

RATIONALE: *Awareness of potential complications produces prompt reporting and immediate intervention.*

OTHER LESS COMMON NURSING DIAGNOSES: *Impaired Tissue Integrity; Altered Tissue Perfusion (peripheral); Potential Altered Urinary Elimination*

ESSENTIAL DISCHARGE CRITERIA

- Shows no active bleeding from circumcision site
- Has no foul odor, pus, or drainage at circumcision site
- Parents demonstrate appropriate skills in care of circumcision
- Circumcision site shows evidence of healing

FAMILY TRANSITION, INFANT INTEGRATION

NURSING DIAGNOSES	OUTCOME CRITERIA	INTERVENTIONS
1 High Risk for Altered Parenting *r.t. lack of knowledge, ineffective role model, lack of support from significant others, interruption of bonding process, unrealistic expectations of infant, presence of stress*	• Risk factors are identified early	• Ascertain if risk factors predisposing to difficulties in parenting exist - review prenatal and intrapartal records for signs of prenatal attachment - note maternal history of chemical dependency - determine feelings about the pregnancy - determine prior involvement with social services, previous history of abuse, and if previous children born to mother are in her care
	• Demonstrates attachment behaviors during parent-infant interactions	• Promote attachment with healthy newborn - keep infant with parents after birth when possible - facilitate breastfeeding within the first 30-60 min of birth - encourage parents to hold, touch, examine, and talk to the infant in the delivery room - provide pain relief for mother - provide rooming in or promote mother-baby/single room maternity care strategies - permit father or significant other to sleep in room with mother - discuss neonate's physical examination and routine care with parents - assist parents to participate in infant care - assist parents in identifying the behavioral capabilities of their infant - encourage bottle-feeding parent to hold infant during feeding

NURSING DIAGNOSES	OUTCOME CRITERIA	INTERVENTIONS
	• Demonstrates attachment behaviors during parent-infant interactions within limitations imposed by illness	• Promote attachment with the ill newborn - encourage parents to see and touch prior to transfer/transport - take Polaroid picture of infant to leave with parents prior to transfer/transport - encourage parents to visit infant transferred to another unit/hospital - explain anticipated equipment used to support sick neonate - inform parents of care given infant - inform parents of infant approach/avoidance behaviors - reinforce normal aspects of infant with a defect
	• Parents/infant show increased quantity and quality of attachment behaviors	• Monitor parent-infant interactions • Reinforce positive parenting behaviors; assist with problem-solving as indicated • Provide follow-up, phone call to determine how family is coping with transition to home • Provide information about parenting groups • Provide referrals to community agencies as needed
		RATIONALE: *Being familiar with an infant's progress and condition helps parents cope and promotes bonding.*
2 Knowledge Deficit (infant care, infant behavior) *r.t. lack of exposure, lack of recall*	• Parents demonstrate knowledge of infant care	• Assess parental teaching needs regarding infant care including - parity and infant care experience - perceptions of parenting behaviors - role priorities as stated - parental expectations related to self and infant - stated knowledge deficit - education
	• Parents demonstrate safe bathing, handling, and inspection techniques	• Instruct parents about infant care including bathing, handling of newborn, detection of symptoms that require medical attention

NURSING DIAGNOSES	OUTCOME CRITERIA	INTERVENTIONS
	• Parents discuss infant feeding and nutrition; ask questions that reflect understanding	• Provide information about newborn's nutritional needs • Instruct about breastfeeding or formula selection, preparation, and storage as indicated • Caution about using microwave to warm formula/breast milk • Instruct parents about fluoride supplementation, vitamins
	• Parents discuss external and internal safety precautions	• Provide information about the proper use of car seat; how to select and use baby equipment appropriately • Assist parents in learning to take infant's temperature • Inform parents of the importance of regular child healthcare and immunizations; discuss symptoms
	• Parents respond appropriately to infant cues	• Demonstrate and discuss infant's capability for interaction • Explain/demonstrate infant status • Discuss importance of determining infant status prior to feeding and other caregiving activities • Assist parents to identify and interpret infant's cues • Demonstrate quieting techniques and ways to increase infant alertness • Point out cues that demonstrate infant responsiveness to parents • Monitor parent's skill in recognizing infant's physiologic needs and performing tasks • Encourage parents to provide auditory, visual, and tactile stimulation • Refer to child care/parenting class • Provide a positive learning environment; encourage parents to ask questions to clarify information

NURSING DIAGNOSES	OUTCOME CRITERIA	INTERVENTIONS
		RATIONALE: *Assessment of parents' skill levels provides a base for a teaching plan commensurate with their abilities.*
3 Anxiety *r.t. change in role functioning, change in environment, maturational crisis*	• Parents identify realistic changes in roles	• Provide for family and sibling visitation during postpartum period • Determine sibling reaction to newborn • Provide information on measures to assist sibling to feel important to the family • Provide information on dealing with sibling rivalry • Provide anticipatory guidance on child development, sleep patterns, and elimination patterns • Assist parents in anticipating safety hazards in the home
		RATIONALE: *Information maximizes parental understanding of normal sibling behavior and allays parental anxiety.*
4 Fatigue *r.t. excessive role demands*	• Assigns priorities to activities; establishes realistic goals; increases activities as endurance builds	• Limit visiting hours to promote rest for mother • Reduce interruptions by hospital personnel • Provide assistance in self-care to maximize focus on infant • Encourage mother to nap when infant sleeping
		RATIONALE: *Role changes and increased responsibilities cause stress for a new mother adapting to physiologic changes postpartum.*

OTHER LESS COMMON NURSING DIAGNOSES: *Altered Role Performance; High Risk for Caregiver Role Strain; Sleep Pattern Disturbance; Ineffective Individual Coping*

ESSENTIAL DISCHARGE CRITERIA

- Is able to care for infant
- Demonstrates attachment behaviors
- Parents verbalize plan for infant follow-up

HEALTHY NEWBORN

NURSING DIAGNOSES	OUTCOME CRITERIA	INTERVENTIONS
1 Ineffective Airway Clearance *r.t. mucus, blood, amniotic fluids swallowed during birth*	• Maintains patent airway - lusty cry - no cyanosis	• Suction OPH, NPH with bulb syringe • Assess needs for gastric decompression/lavage
		RATIONALE: *Regurgitation of gastric contents places infant at risk for aspiration.*
2 Ineffective Breathing Pattern *r.t. transient alteration in chest expansion, immature neurologic controls*	• Shows respiratory status WNL - 40-60 breaths/min • Shows only transitory rhonchi, crackles, irregular breathing, tachypnea, slight sternal retraction	• Monitor respiratory status q15 min until stable then q2-4h as required • Auscultate breath sounds per unit standards • Promote oxygenation, fluid drainage - position on side - keep 0_2 readily available; administer as required
		RATIONALE: *Lung fluid absorption takes 12–72 h.*
3 Ineffective Thermo-regulation *r.t. environmental cooling, immaturity, absence of body fat (SGA, IUGR)*	• Maintains body temperature WNL, stable within 4h after birth	• Assess temperatures immediately after birth, then q15 min to 2h until stable, then q4-8h until discharge
	• Exhibits no evidence of cold stress - no pallor, cyanosis - cry is not feeble - respirations not slow, shallow - no expiratory grunt - no flaccidity - reflexes not slow - no evidence of poor sucking, feeding	• Monitor for s/s of cold stress q15 min-1 h until stable; prevent cold stress - keep nursery/mother's room temperature at required levels - towel-dry infant immediately after birth; wrap in warmed blanket; place on warmed surface - allow mother to cuddle infant to provide warmth - place under radiant warmer if temperature drops - place cap on dry head - postpone bathing until 4 h after delivery, or when temperature is stable
	• Mother discusses need to preserve body warmth of infant	• Explain need to preserve warmth of infant; how to dress, cap, wrap, cuddle, breastfeed

NURSING DIAGNOSES	OUTCOME CRITERIA	INTERVENTIONS
	• Mother demonstrates ability to safely, accurately take temperature	• Demonstrate, explain how to take temperature, read thermometer, analyze findings
		RATIONALE: *Hypothermia places the infant at risk for hypoglycemia, apnea, and acidosis, among other problems.*
4 Altered Nutrition: Less than body requirements *r.t. increased caloric requirement associated with increased metabolic rate*	• Maintains stable or increasing body weight (weight loss for Days 1 and 2 < 10% BW)	• On admission to nursery, weigh, measure, calculate caloric needs
	• Maintains glucose level > 40, < 180 mg/dL	• Perform blood glucose assessment per unit standard protocol; if low, follow with glucose supplement
	• Has normal bowel sounds by 6 h post delivery; passage of meconium by 24-48 h post delivery	• Auscultate bowel sounds, observe for meconium passage
	• Takes, retains 100-200 cal/kg per day	• Assist to establish a regular feeding schedule - initiate breastfeeding as infant stability established - offer feedings per demand or according to recommended schedule - place on right side post feedings to facilitate gastric emptying
	• Shows no evidence of poor feeding - no regurgitation, choking, fatigue during feedings - normal gag and swallowing reflexes - no irritability, dyspnea during feedings	• Assess for s/s of feeding problems: regurgitation, choking, fatigue, irritability, dyspnea
	• Stool colors follow expected patterns - bottle-fed: greenish meconium to yellow-brown and light yellow - breast-fed: greenish meconium to yellow-mustard to pasty	• Assess stools: colors, frequency, characteristics - report clay colored and absence of stool and/or meconium plug
		RATIONALE: *Establishing a feeding pattern is essential. Assist mother to identify feeding duration and/or volume required.*

NURSING DIAGNOSES	OUTCOME CRITERIA	INTERVENTIONS
5 High Risk for Fluid Volume Deficit *r.t. immature kidney function; sensible, insensible fluid losses*	• Maintains balanced I&O - first voiding occurs within 24 h post delivery - urine output WNL - no weight loss after Day 2 - no diarrheal stools	• Monitor I&O q4-8h - assess, document voiding patterns - weigh daily - inspect stools for diarrhea • Offer fluids according to protocol or per orders • Encourage breastfeeding q2-4h while awake
	• Is well hydrated - moist mucous membranes, good skin turgor - normal fontanel tension	• Monitor hydration - inspect mucous membranes, skin - inspect fontanels for tension q4-8h
		RATIONALE: *Adequate fluid balance reflects newborn's health state.*
6 Impaired Skin Integrity *r.t. loss of acid mantle, chemical substances, excretions*	• Displays no rashes, excoriation, skin breaks, lesions	• Examine, protect integumentary mantle - inspect bony prominences and skin for rashes, breaks, lesions q4h - minimize use of tape on skin - use low alkaline soap - limit bathing first few days to preserve acid mantle
		RATIONALE: *Intact skin is first line of defense against infection.*
7 High Risk for Infection *r.t. nosocomial, other bacterial invasion*	• Remains afebrile	• Monitor body temperature q4-8h, or as indicated
	• Displays no skin breaks, rashes, lesions; no redness, drainage, foul odor from cord, circumcision	• Inspect skin, cord, circumcision q8h • Apply bacteriostatic ointment as ordered
	• Shows no evidence of general infection - fever, lethargy, poor feeding - apnea, tachypnea - hypothermia - hypotension, hypotonia - irritability, hypertonia - jaundice, vomiting	• Assess, report presence of any s/s of general infection q8h

NURSING DIAGNOSES	OUTCOME CRITERIA	INTERVENTIONS
	• Experiences benefit of isolation procedure as indicated	• Initiate, maintain required exclusion, protection - handle infant with gloves until first bath - exclude infants with infection or suspected infection from general nursery - handle infants with rashes, skin breaks with sterile gloves only - exclude personnel, family with infections - maintain strict hand-washing
	• Mother/parents discuss concept of bacterial transmission - describe safe behaviors of hand-washing, kissing, protection from infected others	• Explain bacterial transmission, safe behaviors - observe careful hand-washing - protect from infected others
		RATIONALE: *Newborns have increased risk for infection until antibody production begins at 3 months of age.*
8 High Risk for Injury (neurologic) *r.t. metabolic, chemical tissue damage*	• Shows bilirubin, glucose, serum Ca WNL	• Perform heel-stick or capillary blood test for bilirubin, glucose; report deviations
	• Shows PKU test negative; thyroid function WNL	• Perform screening tests for PKU, hypothyroidism • Provide information for follow-up testing
	• Shows negative toxicology screen	• Perform drug screen per institutional protocol
		RATIONALE: *Early identification of metabolic and other potential problems enhances outcome.*

NURSING DIAGNOSES	OUTCOME CRITERIA	INTERVENTIONS
9 Knowledge Deficit *r.t. infant care*	• Mother/parents express feelings about infant care; demonstrate bathing, dressing, feeding, holding, cord and circumcision care	• Provide teaching-learning experiences - identify level of knowledge - listen to concerns, questions - evaluate appropriateness of questions - ascertain prior experience; teach accordingly - demonstrate bathing, feeding, holding, cord care, circumcision care
	• Mother/parents discuss growth and developmental tasks in near future	• Explain, discuss developmental tasks to occur in next month
	• Mother/parents display bonding behaviors; soothes, calms infant	• Assess presence, absence of bonding behaviors; encourage touching, holding, cuddling, talking to infant
	• Mother/parents describe realistic plans for self and infant care	• Discuss required follow-up, well-child care

RATIONALE: *Provide/reinforce essential information to ensure infant safety until first well-baby visit.*

OTHER LESS-COMMON NURSING DIAGNOSES: *Ineffective Breastfeeding; Ineffective Feeding Pattern; Altered Parenting*

ESSENTIAL DISCHARGE CRITERIA

- Maintains balanced I&O; moist membranes, good skin turgor, fontanels not sunken
- Shows < 10% weight loss
- Shows stools following expected pattern for color, amount, frequency for breast or bottle feeding
- Feeds enthusiastically without undue stopping, regurgitating, dyspnea, choking, fatigue
- Displays clear, intact skin; cord, circumcision free of drainage, erythema, foul odor
- Exhibits no s/s of general infection
- Has screening tests completed for bilirubin, glucose, Hb, thyroid, PKU
- Parents discuss feelings about infant care; ask appropriate questions; perform required infant care techniques: bathing, feeding, dressing, diapering, holding, rocking
- Parents demonstrate cord, circumcision care
- Mother displays successful soothing, calming behaviors; parents display normal bonding behaviors
- Parents have follow-up appointment for well-child care

PHYSIOLOGIC JAUNDICE

NURSING DIAGNOSES	OUTCOME CRITERIA	INTERVENTIONS
1 High Risk for Injury *r.t. excessive levels of bilirubin and complications of phototherapy*	• At-risk neonate is identified early	• Identify neonates at risk for developing kernicterus (history of acidosis, asphyxia, cold stress, prematurity, treatment with sulfonamides, etc.)
	• Shows bilirubin levels WNL by 7-11 days in term infants that are not bruised or sick (sick, bruised, and premature infants' levels are slower to return to normal)	• Assess neonate's skin color for jaundice with every general assessment at least q4-8h - assess sclera, skin over the forehead and trunk
	• Exhibits no complications of hyperbilirubinemia and phototherapy - no lethargy - no poor feeding - no loss of moro reflex - no respiratory distress - no high pitched cry, convulsions	• Monitor ordered serum bilirubin levels • Assess behaviors that indicate rising levels of bilirubin q4-8h
	• Experiences no negative side effects of phototherapy	• Institute phototherapy if ordered - protect eyes from phototherapy with eye shields insuring that eyes are closed and shields do not slip over nose - inspect eyes for injury with lights off q4-8h; clean matter away gently with sterile water - maintain infant at appropriate distance from lights; turn q2h - monitor number of hours each lamp is used; change lamp at appropriate intervals to maintain effectiveness - maintain NTE

RATIONALE: *Identification of those at risk for complications and assessment of physiological, behavioral, and biochemical parameters fosters timely interventions.*

NURSING DIAGNOSES	OUTCOME CRITERIA	INTERVENTIONS
2 High Risk for Fluid Volume Deficit *r.t. diarrhea and insensible water loss from phototherapy*	• Maintains adequate hydration	• Feed as ordered at least q4h • Offer water as ordered • Monitor hydration status - fluid and nutritional intake - urine and fecal loss - skin turgor - daily weights - serum electrolytes - urinary sp. gr. • Provide skin care to diaper area • Maintain NTE; assess axillary temperature q2h and prn **RATIONALE:** *Adequate hydration enhances bilirubin excretion.*
3 Altered Parenting *r.t. decreased opportunity to relate to infant receiving phototherapy, lack of knowledge regarding physiologic jaundice of newborn*	• Parents demonstrate bonding behavior despite phototherapy; discuss appropriate caregiving based on understanding of physiologic jaundice	• Assess parents' cognitive level for understanding of neonate's condition and needs • Involve in tasks of parenting; give opportunity to feed, bathe, and comfort neonate • Provide information about physiologic jaundice of the newborn; encourage questions; reinforce or clarify information as needed • Teach to assess neonate for increasing bilirubin levels • Discuss home management of mild to moderate physiologic jaundice including frequency/volume of feedings, exposure to sunlight, and follow-up serum testing programs **RATIONALE:** *Assessment of learning needs, provision of information, and opportunity for caregiving promote attachment and appropriate home management.*

OTHER LESS COMMON NURSING DIAGNOSES: *Interrupted Breastfeeding; Knowledge Deficit; Diarrhea*

ESSENTIAL DISCHARGE CRITERIA

- Shows no adverse effects related to physiologic jaundice
- Takes, retains 90% of feedings; shows consistent weight gain
- Parents verbalize plan for follow-up care and list s/s to report to PCP

COMPROMISED NEONATE

COMP NEONATE

CONTENTS

AIR LEAK SYNDROME

NURSING DIAGNOSES	OUTCOME CRITERIA	INTERVENTIONS
1 Impaired Gas Exchange *r.t. presence of PIE, pneumothorax, pneumopericardium, pneumoperitoneum*	• Exhibits adequate gas exchange - VS WNL - CVP WNL - pulse pressure WNL - pulse oximetry saturation WNL	• Assess and document HR, BP, RR, and pulse oximetry q1-2h and prn • Provide continuous cardiopulmonary monitoring
	• Maintains clear and equal breath sounds bilaterally • Displays symmetrical chest expansion; PMI at 5-6 intercostal space, midclavicular line; clear heart tones	• Auscultate breath and heart sounds q2-4h - monitor chest expansion and PMI location - have needle aspiration kit at bedside
	• Shows no s/s of respiratory distress such as - no agitation - no retractions - no nasal flaring - no grunting, gasping - no cyanosis/pallor - no abnormal blood gas	• Monitor for respiratory distress • Position to maintain open airway - elevate HOB 30-40° • Administer O_2 as ordered • Maintain suction set-up • Monitor blood gases
		RATIONALE: *Prompt recognition of early s/s of air leak syndrome permits early intervention to prevent acute deterioration and complications.*
2 Decreased Cardiac Output *r.t. pneumothorax, pneumopericardium, pneumoperitoneum*	• Exhibits adequate C.O. - VS WNL - CVP WNL - LOC WNL - strong/equal peripheral pulses - CRT < 3 sec - sufficient urinary output 0.5-3 mL/kg/h - sp. gr. 1.005-1.020	• Assess and document HR, BP q1-2h and prn, or place on continuous cardiopulmonary monitor • Maintain patent IV • Assess LOC; monitor for agitation • Administer O_2 • Assess CRT and peripheral pulses q1-2h and prn • Maintain accurate I&O • Monitor urinary sp. gr.
	• Maintains adequate C.O. through interventions necessary to relieve air leak	• Have needle aspiration kit at bedside • Anticipate need for chest tube insertion

NURSING DIAGNOSES	OUTCOME CRITERIA	INTERVENTIONS
		• If needle aspiration performed - document infant's response to procedure - document amount of air or fluid removed - administer O_2 to keep saturation within parameters - place occlusive pressure dressing on site - assess need for pain medication • If chest tube inserted - premedicate as ordered - secure chest tube to body and to bed to prevent traction on tube - keep padded hemostat at bedside - keep occlusive dressing at bedside - document infant's response to procedure - administer O_2 to keep O_2 sats within parameters - assess need for pain medication • Monitor chest tube drainage system - tape all connections - set pressure and suction - mark drainage level q shift - document drainage and amount q4h - monitor bubbling at least qh
		RATIONALE: *Timely assessment and early intervention to maintain C.O. will maintain perfusion to vital organs.*
3 High Risk for Injury *r.t. procedures necessary to relieve air leak*	• Tolerates procedures - VS returning to baseline - no untoward effects	• Medicate infant to lower anxiety and fighting during procedure • Administer O_2 as ordered • Maintain airway; have artificial airway and intubation set up at bedside • Restrain as necessary with soft restraints during procedure
		RATIONALE: *Preplanning for potential complications allows for quicker responses and access to necessary equipment.*

OTHER LESS COMMON NURSING DIAGNOSES: *Pain; High Risk for Infection; High Risk for Altered Parenting*

ESSENTIAL DISCHARGE CRITERIA

- Air leak is resolved
- Maintains adequate ventilation without support

ANEMIA

NURSING DIAGNOSES	OUTCOME CRITERIA	INTERVENTIONS
1 High Risk for Infection *r.t. decreased resistance secondary to tissue hypoxia*	• Experiences no infection secondary to tissue hypoxia	• Identify risk factors • Assess condition, noting s/s of infection q1-2h
	• Exhibits stable VS	• Assess pulse, VS q2-4h; assess BP q4-8h
	• Shows normal CBC, ABGs	• Monitor CBC, Hct/reticulocyte count q day - administer blood per orders - observe for transfusion reactions • Monitor ABGs
	• Shows normal tissue perfusion - pulses 2+ - CRT < 3 sec - has pink mucous membranes	• Assess tissue perfusion q2-4h
		RATIONALE: *Decreasing tissue O_2 consumption requirements reduces the risk of infection. Careful monitoring for s/s of infection allows for early detection and treatment of infection.*
2 Activity Intolerance *r.t. impaired O_2 transport secondary to diminished RBC count*	• Exhibits normal infant activity level - is alert with feedings - has lusty cry - tolerates care/handling	• Cluster nursing care activities • Increase O_2 prn with caregiving and/or procedures as indicated by VS/pulse or history • Provide comfort measures prn • Evaluate lab work per orders; note CBC, Hct • Give blood products per orders • Be alert to signs of stress and delay procedures if necessary
		RATIONALE: *Activity intolerance is minimized when care is organized to allow for rest periods. O_2 and blood products increase RBC capacity.*

OTHER LESS COMMON NURSING DIAGNOSES: *Altered Tissue Perfusion; High Risk for Injury (bleeding); Impaired Gas Exchange*

ESSENTIAL DISCHARGE CRITERIA

- Shows no s/s of infection; has normal CBC, VS
- Tolerates normal activity without O_2
- Takes, retains 90% of feedings
- Parents verbalize s/s of infant stress and plan to report to PCP

APNEA OF PREMATURITY

NURSING DIAGNOSES	OUTCOME CRITERIA	INTERVENTIONS
1 Ineffective Breathing Pattern *r.t. apneic episodes*	• RR is WNL • Has clear and equal breath sounds	• Assess respiration q2-4h and prn - RR, depth, rhythm - quality of breath sounds - presence/absence of s/s of distress
	• Shows VS WNL	• Provide cardiopulmonary monitoring as ordered - low HR alarm and apnea delay set per unit standard • Keep emergency equipment available at all times - resuscitation bag and mask - O_2 - suction
	• Exhibits no cyanosis, grunting, retractions, nasal flaring	• Document apneic episodes, include - state of infant at time of episode (asleep, awake, feeding) - physiologic changes during episode - interventions needed to initiate respirations • Administer medications as ordered - monitor blood levels as ordered
	• Shows blood gas values within acceptable range for infant	• Monitor blood gas values; report to physician
		RATIONALE: *Rapid response to apneic episodes minimizes hypoxia and the potential for periventricular leukomalacia.*
2 Anxiety *r.t. apneic episodes*	• Parents verbalize/demonstrate understanding of diagnosis	• Assess parents' understanding of apnea, implications for infant • Complete teaching as needed - diagnosis - equipment - treatments/tests - medications
	• Parents display effective coping strategies	• Assess and facilitate parents' coping responses, i.e., verbalization, behavior, caregiving

NURSING DIAGNOSES	OUTCOME CRITERIA	INTERVENTIONS
	• Parents express, display increased emotional comfort	• Provide support to parents as needed - encourage verbalization of concerns and questions - answer questions honestly - initiate referral to outside resources as appropriate
		RATIONALE: *Education and emotional support can reduce anxiety.*
3 Knowledge Deficit *r.t. apnea monitoring, home care*	• Parents verbalize/demonstrate - understanding of diagnosis, treatments, medications - use/care of home monitor	• Assess parents' understanding of home care needs for the infant on a monitor • Complete or refer teaching as needed, including - diagnosis - treatments - medications - use/care of home monitor
	• Parents demonstrate required skills for intervention in apneic episode	• Explain care of infant during apneic episode - stimulation - CPR - emergency phone numbers - record of apneic episodes
	• Parents affirm importance of follow-up with PCP and other identified resources	• Discuss need for routine visits to PCP • Complete appropriate community referrals
		RATIONALE: *This teaching prepares parents to provide safe care for infant at home.*

OTHER LESS COMMON NURSING DIAGNOSES: *High Risk for Impaired Skin Integrity; High Risk for Caregiver Role Strain; Inability to Sustain Spontaneous Ventilation*

ESSENTIAL DISCHARGE CRITERIA

- Blood gases WNL
- Homegoing medications are at therapeutic levels
- Apnea episodes respond to tactile stimulation
- Parents demonstrate ability to care for infant, including monitoring and CPR
- Parents possess emergency phone numbers and follow-up appointments

ASPHYXIA

NURSING DIAGNOSES	OUTCOME CRITERIA	INTERVENTIONS
1 Impaired Gas Exchange *r.t. pulmonary arteriolar constriction, increased pulmonary vascular resistance, decreased pulmonary blood flow, CNS compromise*	• Exhibits adequate gas exchange - normal blood gases - PCO_2 levels at lower limits of normal - pH levels at higher limits of normal	• Monitor blood gases as ordered • Assess continuous pulse oximetry/transcutaneous O_2 monitoring • Adjust inspired O_2 within ordered parameters • Notify physician of trends
	• Exhibits no CNS compromise - respirations 40-60 bpm - no apnea - no bradycardia	• Assess VS hourly or as indicated • Provide continuous cardiopulmonary monitoring
		RATIONALE: *Adequate oxygenation facilitates physiologic stability.*
2 Decreased Cardiac Output *r.t. pulmonary edema; pulmonary arteriolar constriction; shift to interstitial space*	• Has normal VS, BP - regular HR	• Provide continuous cardiopulmonary monitoring • Assess VS, BP qh and as indicated
	• Shows adequate peripheral circulation - CRT < 3 sec - no mottling - strong pulses	• Assess tissue perfusion q2-4h • Assess peripheral pulses q4h • Administer IV fluids and vasodilators as ordered
	• Exhibits normal circulating volume - balanced I&O - normal urine output - normal CVP	• Monitor I&O; weigh all diapers • Assess CVP, BP qh • Administer volume expanders as ordered
		RATIONALE: *Asphyxia can damage the cardiac muscle causing altered cardiac output, which leads to problems with tissue perfusion. Fluid shift to the interstitial space decreases circulating volume. Adequate tissue perfusion provides O_2 and nutrition to enable cellular functions.*

NURSING DIAGNOSES	OUTCOME CRITERIA	INTERVENTIONS
3 Activity Intolerance *r.t. CNS irritability*	• Exhibits no desaturations or bradycardia	• Provide minimal stimulation environment • Provide continuous cardiopulmonary monitoring, respond to alarms promptly
	• Quiets with caregiver support	• Minimize conversation at bedside • Hang "quiet" sign • Cluster care as tolerated • Dim lights or darken room as appropriate • Minimize handling of infant • Record VS off monitor • Use prone or side-lying positioning as indicated • Administer analgesics as indicated
	• Maintains position of comfort	• Nest infant, provide containment • Provide sheepskin, gel pillow, wedge
		RATIONALE: *The NICU environment is overstimulating, especially for very sick infants. Infant physiologic responses may place added compromise on the neonate's system.*
4 Altered Renal Tissue Perfusion *r.t. hypovolemia, ischemia*	• Maintains normal output	• Maintain strict I&O; weigh diapers • Administer diuretics as ordered
	• Shows normal urine chemistries	• Monitor urine lab work • Perform urine dip for protein, glucose, electrolytes, RBC
	• Shows normal blood chemistries - experiences normal peak and trough levels	• Monitor blood chemistries • Administer nephrotoxic medications (gentamicin) with care
		RATIONALE: *During an asphyxial event, blood is shunted away from the kidneys to vital organs, increasing the potential for ischemia.*

NURSING DIAGNOSES	OUTCOME CRITERIA	INTERVENTIONS
5 High Risk for Infection *r.t. nosocomial invasion, compromised immune response, debilitation*	• Exhibits no s/s of systemic infection - no signs of sepsis - no apnea, dyspnea - no thermal instability - no pallor, cyanosis	• Assess parameters and provide interventions to support infant - perform continuous cardiopulmonary monitoring - provide thermal support
	• Has normal CBC for gestation	• Monitor blood counts
	• Experiences normal peak and trough levels	• Administer antibiotics as ordered • Monitor peak and trough levels
		RATIONALE: *The neonate is at increased risk for infection. Asphyxia may be the result of an infectious process. Multiple IV lines increase the risk of nosocomial infection.*
6 Knowledge Deficit *r.t. disease process, potential sequelae/death of neonate, interruption of bonding process*	• Parents verbalize understanding of treatment plan	• Provide information - explain disease process - assess coping skills - link with peer support group - provide ongoing updates re progress
	• Parents provide care for infant	• Teach parents approach/avoidance signals • Teach parents specialized care
	• Parents verbalize/demonstrate taking in of infant into family	• Promote attachment through role modeling and family trait identification
		RATIONALE: *Life-threatening illness places the family at risk for multiple challenges. Communication is essential. Information and role modeling will facilitate the family's taking in of the neonate.*

OTHER LESS COMMON NURSING DIAGNOSES: *Altered Nutrition: Less than body requirements; Ineffective Thermoregulation; Inability to Sustain Spontaneous Ventilation; Anticipatory Grieving; Ineffective Breathing Pattern; Altered Tissue Perfusion; Ineffective Infant Feeding Pattern*

ESSENTIAL DISCHARGE CRITERIA

- Takes, retains 90% of feedings; shows consistent weight gain
- Has balanced I&O
- Parents demonstrate skill in performing required care
- Parents list s/s to be reported to PCP

ASSISTED VENTILATION

NURSING DIAGNOSES	OUTCOME CRITERIA	INTERVENTIONS
1 Impaired Gas Exchange *r.t. ventilation perfusion imbalance, decreased energy/fatigue*	• Exhibits VS WNL for infant - RR, HR WNL - color pink - BP, CVP WNL • Has clear and equal breath sounds • Has mild to absent retractions • Has no grunting, nasal flaring, cyanosis	• Provide continuous cardiopulmonary monitoring • Assess and record q1-2h and prn - VS including RR, depth, rhythm, use of accessory muscles - HR, BP - quality of breath sounds - chest excursion - color - presence/absence of grunting, nasal flaring, retractions - ventilator settings - bilateral air entry
	• Shows blood gas values within acceptable range for patient	• Monitor and report blood gas values to physician • Provide transcutaneous monitoring and/or pulse oximetry as ordered
	• Shows symmetrical chest rise without over expansion	• Ensure ventilator setting changes are made as ordered • Maintain patent airway, suction prn • Report any sudden deterioration in VS/infant's condition • Elevate HOB • Coordinate respiratory therapy/nursing care to facilitate accuracy of blood gases • Assess need for NG or OG suction to relieve gastric distention • Note decompensation; intervene and note - precipitating events - agitation - frequent suctioning - low Hb - positioning • Provide comfort measures prn • Give sedation if ordered • Plan for rest periods

RATIONALE: *Monitoring prompts early detection of respiratory compromise.*

COMP NEONATE

NURSING DIAGNOSES	OUTCOME CRITERIA	INTERVENTIONS
2 Ineffective Airway Clearance *r.t. tracheobronchial secretions*	• Has clear airway - has clear and equal breath sounds - shows no increased work of breathing - has mild to absent retractions	• Assess breath sounds q1-2h and prn • Increase FiO_2 by 10% or higher as needed before suctioning • Suction as needed - measure length of ETT to determine appropriate depth for suctioning; note depth on bedside card - suction pressure 80-100 mmHg - instill sterile saline as needed for very thick secretions - apply intermittent suction as catheter is withdrawn from ETT • Document quality of secretions, infant's tolerance of procedures • Provide chest physiotherapy as ordered • Have standby ETT at bedside • Ensure that ETT is secured to patient at all times; record ETT position (i.e., marking at lip) • Use nesting to contain infant, prevent agitation • Reposition q2-4h unless contraindicated • Maintain humidity to ventilator
		RATIONALE: *These interventions mobilize secretions and maintain a patent airway, promoting adequate gas exchange.*
3 High Risk for Infection *r.t. immature immune system, invasive procedures*	• Exhibits normal temperature, VS	• Assess temperature, pulse, respiration qh; notify physician of temp > 38°C (100.4°F)
	• Shows WBC count WNL	• Monitor/report lab values as ordered
	• Shows normal tracheal secretions (no thick or yellow secretions)	• Observe/report changes in quality of tracheal secretions • Maintain sterile technique during ET suctioning • Cover infant's eyes when suctioning to prevent splashing of tracheal secretions

NURSING DIAGNOSES	OUTCOME CRITERIA	INTERVENTIONS
		RATIONALE: *Maintaining sterile technique minimizes risk of infection; diligent monitoring allows prompt recognition of infectious processes.*

OTHER LESS COMMON NURSING DIAGNOSES: *Decreased Cardiac Output; Dysfunctional Ventilatory Weaning Response; Impaired Skin Integrity; Ineffective Infant Feeding Pattern; High Risk for Injury; Ineffective Breathing Pattern*

ESSENTIAL DISCHARGE CRITERIA

- Sustains spontaneous respirations without assisted ventilation
- Shows blood gases WNR for patient
- Requires minimal to no supplemental O_2
- Has clear and equal breath sounds

BEHAVIORAL-BASED CARE

NURSING DIAGNOSES	OUTCOME CRITERIA	INTERVENTIONS
1 Activity Intolerance *r.t. disease process, prematurity, multiple procedures*	• Remains physiologically organized during interventions	• Assess for approach/avoidance behaviors before, during, and after to intervention • Cluster care as tolerated by infant • Provide containment during turning • Provide non-nutritive sucking as comfort measure • Minimize extraneous environmental stimulation
	• Maintains regular HR/RR • Maintains O_2 sats WNL (as indicated by disease process)	• Provide continuous cardiopulmonary/pulse oximetry monitoring • Assess HR, RR q2-4h • Trend data to identify problematic interventions/times of day
		RATIONALE: *Attention to infant behaviors will indicate tolerance of interventions/activities.*
2 Sleep Pattern Disturbance *r.t. environment, interventions, pharmacologics*	• Attains deep sleep	• Minimize environmental stimulation during States 1 and 2 • Cover isolette with blankets • Shield face from light • Dim lights as appropriate
	• Demonstrates consistent weight gain	• Organize care to promote establishment of predictable biorhythms • Establish medication schedule to minimize impact on sleep cycle, i.e., theophylline • Teach family importance of deep sleep and strategies to promote this state
		RATIONALE: *Neonates maximize calorie utilization for weight gain during deep sleep (State 1).*

NURSING DIAGNOSES	OUTCOME CRITERIA	INTERVENTIONS
3 Sensory/ Perceptual Alterations *r.t. immaturity, medications, position change limitations, excessive environmental stimuli*	• Quiets to auditory stimulation	• Assess appropriateness of, and provide, auditory stimulation - music box - taped parent voices, music, stories, heartbeat - soft vocalizations
	• Shows HR/RR stable while attending to visual stimuli	• Assess appropriateness of, and provide, visual stimulation - en face position - black-and-white patterns - pictures - mobile • Provide single item in visual field, initially
	• Retains tone and state	• Assess appropriateness of, and provide, tactile/kinesthetic stimulation - rock infant - massage
		RATIONALE: *Developmentally appropriate interventions provide the infant with opportunities to continue normal maturation of the CNS.*
4 Impaired Physical Mobility *r.t. limited range of motion, decreased muscle strength, immaturity*	• Maintains range of motion in all joints; has no contractures	• Position infant in anatomically correct position
	• Maintains flexion, centering of limbs	• Use devices to minimize shoulder extension - gel pillow - doughnut - hip rolls - nesting - containment - wedge/blanket rolls • Provide sheepskin
	• Demonstrates smooth, coordinated movements appropriate to gestational age	• Assess need for ROM exercises, perform as indicated and infant tolerates - instruct, encourage parents to perform

NURSING DIAGNOSES	OUTCOME CRITERIA	INTERVENTIONS
		RATIONALE: *Acute illness may additionally compromise the neonate's ability to retain muscle mass and ROM.*

OTHER LESS COMMON NURSING DIAGNOSES: *Altered Growth and Development; Knowledge Deficit; Ineffective Infant Feeding Pattern; Fatigue*

ESSENTIAL DISCHARGE CRITERIA

- Is physiologically stable when stressed, integrates environmental stimuli
- Sleep-wake pattern is established
- Parents demonstrate behavioral/developmental concept integration into interactions with infant

BOWEL OBSTRUCTION

NURSING DIAGNOSES	OUTCOME CRITERIA	INTERVENTIONS
1 High Risk for Fluid Volume Deficit *r.t. vomiting, hypermetabolic state, NPO status*	• Exhibits fluids and electrolytes WNL - balanced I&O - weight loss WNL - urinary sp. gr. WNL	• Weigh at same time each day • Administer IV fluids as ordered by physician • Monitor elecctrolyte studies • Monitor I&O hourly, report deviations • Monitor urinary sp. gr.
		RATIONALE: *Fluid and electrolyte balance must be maintained to prevent dehydration.*
2 High Risk for Infection *r.t. inadequate primary defenses, surgical intervention, open wound (ostomy)*	• Body temperature WNL	• Assess vital signs, especially temperature as indicated q2h, report temperature > 38°C (100.4°F)
	• Shows soft, nontense abdomen, no loops of bowel - surgical incision clean, dry, intact - ostomy mucosa pink, moist	• Assess abdomen/incision for s/s of infection (erythema, warmth, purulent discharge) • Change dressing as indicated using sterile techniques • Teach child and family s/s of infection and home care of incision • Administer antibiotics as ordered
		RATIONALE: *Early identification of infection minimizes surgical complications.*
3 Pain *r.t. obstruction, surgical procedure*	• Shows no pain or reduction in pain	• Assess for presence of pain - irritability - tachycardia - guarding • Assess the family for the presence of misconceptions about pain and its treatment • Make child as comfortable as possible - provide analgesics as ordered by physician - respond immediately to signs of pain - use nonpharmacologic techniques to reduce pain

NURSING DIAGNOSES	OUTCOME CRITERIA	INTERVENTIONS
		• Notify physician of ineffective pain management, changes in type, level, location of pain
		RATIONALE: *Increase child's comfort by decreasing level of pain; use presence of pain as an indication of a change in condition.*
4 Knowledge Deficit *r.t. lack of experience*	• Parents/family verbalize understanding of current illness and its treatment and implications for home care	• Assess family's knowledge of current illness and its treatment • Encourage parents to ask questions • Establish mutual goals for the care of the child • Reinforce physician's information about child's treatment and surgical procedure, if indicated • Provide post-op and home care information • Provide consultation referrals as needed
		RATIONALE: *Parents who are informed about their child's condition experience less stress and provide appropriate care.*

OTHER LESS COMMON NURSING DIAGNOSES: *High Risk for Altered Parenting; Ineffective Breathing Patterns; Altered Tissue Perfusion; Nutrition: Less than body requirements; Anxiety (parents); High Risk for Injury*

ESSENTIAL DISCHARGE CRITERIA

- Bowel sounds are present; no abdominal distension
- Incision is without s/s of infection
- Shows consistent weight gain
- Takes, retains 90% of prescribed nutrition, fluids
- Parents demonstrate required care techniques
- Parents possess follow-up appointments

CHEMICAL ADDICTION/WITHDRAWAL

NURSING DIAGNOSES	OUTCOME CRITERIA	INTERVENTIONS
1 Ineffective Infant Feeding Pattern *r.t. neurologic impairment, oral hypersensitivity*	• Sustain effective suck and coordinates sucking, swallowing, and breathing	• Assess infant's suck, swallow, breathing coordination • Use pacifier to satisfy non-nutritive sucking needs
	• Retains 90% of feedings	• Decrease feeding intervals to allow for frequent, small feedings • Provide nasogastric/orogastric feeds when indicated by prolonged feeding time, disorganized suck, need for rest • Observe amount of gastric aspirates before feeding if nasogastric/orogastric feedings are used
	• Gains weight	• Consider high calorie formulas or fortified breast milk if indicated • Weigh daily on same scale
	• Parents verbalize understanding of infant's nutritional needs	• Inform parents of rationale for alternative feeding approaches and need for increased nutritional intake during withdrawal period
		RATIONALE: *Infants exposed to drugs may have increased metabolic needs in addition to withdrawal symptoms necessitating alternative nutritional support.*
2 Sleep Pattern Disturbance *r.t. interrupted sleep, changes in behavior, physiologic disturbances*	• Demonstrates sleep pattern appropriate for age	• Assess patterns of sleep and activity • Provide a quiet, darkened environment that allows for observation • Use calming techniques - swaddling - skin-to-skin contact - use of front pack - vertical rocking • Encourage parents/cuddler to hold and comfort infant
		RATIONALE: *Environmental effects impact sleep patterns and produce changes in state-related behavior such as hyperirritability.*

NURSING DIAGNOSES	OUTCOME CRITERIA	INTERVENTIONS
3 High Risk for Impaired Skin Integrity *r.t. mechanical factors, altered metabolic state, physical immobilization, hyperactivity*	• Skin remains intact with no erythema or breakdown	• Assess skin integrity over bony prominences, knees, elbows, cheeks, and perineal area frequently • Change infant's position when alert and after feeding • Use sheepskin under infant • Change diaper soon after elimination; leave perineal area exposed to air as much as possible
		RATIONALE: *Infants experiencing withdrawal may develop rub marks or excoriated buttocks from diarrhea. Interventions promote skin integrity.*
4 Knowledge Deficit *r.t. unfamiliarity with infant's condition*	• Parents explain or demonstrate caregiving activities that maximize infant's comfort, growth, and development	• Assess family's knowledge of withdrawal experiences and relate to infant's condition • Provide parent education and anticipatory guidance regarding infant care, techniques for consoling and feeding, and pharmacologic interventions
	• Parents discuss s/s of complications: excessive crying/ irritability, diaphoresis, irritated skin, dyspnea	• Discuss complications to report
	• Parents express feelings about infant's condition	• Encourage family to discuss their feelings and concerns regarding infant's condition
		RATIONALE: *Educating the parents will assist them to be effective caregivers.*
5 High Risk for Caregiver Role Strain *r.t. premature birth, inexperienced with caregiving, addiction*	• Parents identify useful coping mechanisms in caring for their infant	• Assess the developmental state of parents and availability of support systems • Provide parents opportunities to express fears, anger, and frustration • Facilitate identification of effective and appropriate parenting behaviors

NURSING DIAGNOSES	OUTCOME CRITERIA	INTERVENTIONS
		• Coordinate referrals to appropriate resources, i.e., Public Health Department, Children's Protective Services • Encourage parents to room-in and assume total care for their child prior to discharge **RATIONALE:** *Drug-exposed infants may be difficult to care for and therefore cause feelings of inadequacy for the caregiver.*

OTHER LESS COMMON NURSING DIAGNOSES: *Altered Nutrition: Less than body requirements; Ineffective Breathing Pattern; Pain*

ESSENTIAL DISCHARGE CRITERIA

- Takes, retains 90% of feedings, gains weight
- Is able to coordinate suck, swallow, and breathing
- Parents demonstrate essential care for infant and are able to provide intervention to comfort infant
- Parents verbalize plans for follow-up care

CHRONIC LUNG DISEASE (BRONCHOPULMONARY DYSPLASIA)

NURSING DIAGNOSES	OUTCOME CRITERIA	INTERVENTIONS
1 Impaired Gas Exchange *r.t. alveolar wall and capillary endothelial damage, accumulation of exudate and cellular debris in small airways, altered mucociliary function*	• Shows oxygenation, ventilation WNL - individually appropriate blood gas and ventilatory parameters	• Carefully monitor ventilatory and blood gas parameters, report to PCP as indicated • Evaluate infant's tolerance of these parameters
	• Maintains stable, normal respiratory status - rate, rhythm, depth, and effort of respiration WNL - pink skin, mucous membranes - breath sounds equal bilaterally - calms to comforting measures	• Assess respiratory status q1-3h • Administer bronchodilators and/or steroids as indicated • Monitor for methylxanthine toxicity • Provide appropriate ventilatory support as indicated O_2 therapy, ventilator, physiotherapy, suctioning) • Provide comfort measures as indicated • Evaluate and document response to medications, comfort measures, and other treatments
		RATIONALE: *Avoiding hypoxia and reducing reinjury allows lungs to heal. Promote calming and minimize stress reactions to foster healing.*
2 Fluid Volume Excess (high risk for) *r.t. fluid retention, steroids, altered renal perfusion*	• Demonstrates no symptoms of fluid overload - urine output appropriate - BP stable - no edema - stable behavior - PCO_2 WNL	• Monitor urine output, report as indicated • Administer diuretics as indicated • Monitor weight gain, edema, behavior changes, sp. gr., urine output, BP • Auscultate and assess respiratory status for rate, distress, and PCO_2 on blood gases
	• Shows electrolytes WNL	• Monitor serum electrolytes as indicated once a week
	• Weight gain WNL - 10-20 g/day	• Weigh daily, same scale • Administer restricted fluid therapy as indicated, e.g., increased caloric density of formula

NURSING DIAGNOSES	OUTCOME CRITERIA	INTERVENTIONS
		RATIONALE: *Minimize fluids to avoid fluid overload and reduce pulmonary edema.*
3 Altered Nutrition: Less than body requirements *r.t. increased resting metabolic expenditure, increased O_2 consumption and fluid restriction, maladaptive feeding behaviors, and low stress tolerance*	• Gains weight WNL - retains 90% of feedings	• Provide adequate daily caloric intake as needed (usually 120-150 kcal/kg/day) • Provide non-nutritive sucking and encourage hand-to-mouth motion • Individualize feeding schedule based on infant's own sleep-wake states and routines • Reduce extraneous stimulation during feeding • Provide swaddling and containment • Identify behaviors that indicate stress intolerance • Position infant to prevent gastroesophageal reflux • Increase inspired O_2 during feedings as indicated by pulse oximetry
		RATIONALE: *Maximize caloric intake, minimize caloric expenditures, promote optimal growth and healing, and compensate for increased O_2 and caloric consumption.*
4 Altered Growth and Development *r.t. multiple caretakers, environmental and stimulation excesses and deficiencies, impaired physical mobility, inconsistent responsiveness to infants, separation from parents, low stress tolerance*	• Performs developmental skills appropriate to adjusted age	• Reduce environmental stimuli - allow for periods of uninterrupted sleep by clustering and pacing caregiving - minimize frequency of capillary and venous bloodwork • Assess infant's readiness for interaction and activity; provide development enhancement - rocking - gentle stroking - visual and auditory stimulation with human face and voice - holding • Refer for individualized developmental assessment and intervention (NIDCAP, APIB)

NURSING DIAGNOSES	OUTCOME CRITERIA	INTERVENTIONS
	• Parents identify and respond appropriately to infant's behavioral cues	• Facilitate consistent, collaborative, multidisciplinary caregiving, including parents as team members • Teach parents to assess, identify, and intervene appropriately to infant's behavioral cues • Determine infant tolerance to procedures and individualize care based on infant cues and physiologic responses • Assess and intervene to minimize stress intolerance
		RATIONALE: *Facilitate early detection and intervention of problems; individualized developmental enhancement program can maximize weight gain, respiratory function, and development while minimizing stress; facilitate competency of parents to optimize developmental outcome.*

OTHER LESS COMMON NURSING DIAGNOSIS: *High Risk for Activity Intolerance; High Risk for Decreased Cardiac Output; Ineffective Management of Therapeutic Regimen; High Risk for Caregiver Role Strain; High Risk for Sleep Pattern Disturbance; High Risk for Infection*

ESSENTIAL DISCHARGE CRITERIA

- Maintains stable respiratory status
- Gains weight WNL, takes 90% of feedings
- Parents demonstrate ability to provide complex care for infant
- Parents verbalize importance of healthcare follow-up

CLEFT LIP, CLEFT PALATE

NURSING DIAGNOSES	OUTCOME CRITERIA	INTERVENTIONS
1 High Risk for Altered Nutrition: Less than body requirements *r.t. inability to suck secondary to cleft lip/palate*	• Takes oral nutrients at appropriate volume for age and weight - gains weight: 15-30 g/day	• Offer nipple feedings with soft nipple or special cleft palate nipple/nurser - feed infant with bottle held securely and cheeks grasped - hold infant in an upright or semiupright position - direct flow of milk to side of mouth - burp frequently - offer frequent, small feedings - offer small amount of sterile water after each feeding, as ordered • Support mother through breastfeeding, as appropriate
		RATIONALE: *These measures help infant create necessary vacuum for adequate sucking, avoid excessive air swallowing and choking, and prevent fatigue, frustration.*
2 High Risk for Aspiration *r.t. altered airway*	• Maintains respiratory efforts WNL - breath sounds clear, equal	• Assess breath sounds q4h • Assess respiratory effort q2-4h
	• Shows no choking, emesis, or spitting up	• Provide ready access to suction - bulb in crib with infant at all times • Position with HOB elevated or in infant seat, as indicated • Burp frequently during feeding
		RATIONALE: *The cleft increases communication with the airway, thereby increasing the potential for aspiration.*

OTHER LESS COMMON NURSING DIAGNOSES: *High Risk for Ineffective Management of Therapeutic Regimen; High Risk for Altered Growth and Development*

ESSENTIAL DISCHARGE CRITERIA

- Takes appropriate amount of oral nutrients
- Shows appropriate weight gain
- Parents demonstrate feeding technique that minimizes potential for aspiration
- Appropriate referral and follow-up is documented

COCAINE EXPOSURE

NURSING DIAGNOSES	OUTCOME CRITERIA	INTERVENTIONS
1 Altered Nutrition: Less than body requirements *r.t. feeding problems; uncoordinated or ineffective sucking, swallowing and breathing; diarrhea, vomiting, colic*	• Demonstrates optimal nutritional status - daily weight gain - retains 90% of feedings - electrolytes WNL - balanced I&O	• Monitor and record nutritional intake based on calories and volume • Weigh daily, same scale • Monitor fluid and electrolyte status • Monitor daily I&O • Assess suck and swallow coordination • Utilize fortified formula, supplement breast milk as needed • Initiate gavage feedings when necessary • Give small frequent feedings • Minimize sensory stimuli during feedings • Teach parents/caregivers strategies for effective feedings **RATIONALE:** *Careful feeding prevents complications related to poor nutritional status and overcomes the effects of altered feeding patterns.*
2 Altered Growth and Development *r.t. effects of maternal drug use, neurologic impairment, decreased attentiveness to environmental stimuli*	• Growth and development patterns WNL - achieves optimal neurologic function	• Assess growth and development patterns of infant • Teach parents/caregivers about - normal patterns of growth and development - activities that support growth and development - refer to community intervention program **RATIONALE:** *These measures facilitate maximum potential for growth and development.*

NURSING DIAGNOSES	OUTCOME CRITERIA	INTERVENTIONS
3 Diarrhea *r.t. effects of withdrawal, increased peristalsis secondary to hyperirritability*	• Frequency and consistency of stools WNL	• Observe and record number and consistency of stools each day • Assess abdomen and note bowel sounds • Medicate as ordered
	• Shows balanced electrolytes	• Monitor serum electrolytes • Monitor and record I&O
	• Has good skin turgor	• Assess skin turgor
	• Skin is free of irritation	• Provide peri-care and rectal care as needed
	• Shows adequate weight gain	• Administer food and fluids as ordered • Teach parents/caregivers to seek medical attention if diarrhea persists for more than 24 h • Teach parents/caregivers the signs of dehydration
		RATIONALE: *All of these measures combine to prevent complications related to diarrhea.*
4 High Risk for Impaired Skin Integrity *r.t. G.I. disturbance (diarrhea) or friction rubs (due to hyperactivity)*	• Shows intact, dry skin	• Observe and record skin condition frequently • Refrain from the use of tape when possible • Use mild soap and water when indicated • Change diapers immediately after elimination • Use cloth diapers if sensitive to disposable diapers • Apply protective dressings or ointment as needed • Use sheepskin in crib or isolette
		RATIONALE: *Monitoring and protecting skin are essential for hyperactive infant.*

NURSING DIAGNOSES	OUTCOME CRITERIA	INTERVENTIONS
5 Sleep Pattern Disturbance *r.t. effects of illicit drugs or medications*	• Demonstrates sleep pattern appropriate for age	• Observe infant's sleep pattern • Allow for uninterrupted periods of sleep • Provide swaddling and skin-to-skin contact • Provide a dark, quiet environment
		RATIONALE: *Drug withdrawal often has a hypo- or hypersensitivity to environmental stimulation component.*
6 High Risk for Injury (external) *r.t. increased hyperirritability and the potential for seizure activity*	• Shows decrease in irritability	• Reduce stimuli in nursery environment • Teach parents about safety measures and strategies to reduce irritability
	• Shows no seizure activity	• Administer appropriate medications as ordered • Institute safety measures to protect infant
		RATIONALE: *These protective measures minimize hyperirritability and seizure potential.*
7 Altered Parenting *r.t. substance abuse, impaired or lack of attachment behaviors, inadequate support systems*	• Parents display bonding behaviors	• Assess parents' readiness to bond with infant • Provide early and repeated parent/infant contact • Encourage and reinforce parenting behavior • Document parent/child interaction
	• Parents verbalize, affirm the infant's need for a nurturing environment	• Assess parents' understanding of the need for a nurturing environment • Encourage verbalization about perception of the child and feelings about parenting • Refer to support services and support groups as needed

NURSING DIAGNOSES	OUTCOME CRITERIA	INTERVENTIONS
		RATIONALE: *Ensure that the parents have an understanding of the importance of a nurturing environment.*

OTHER LESS COMMON NURSING DIAGNOSES: *Infection; Sensory Perceptual Alterations: Ineffective Airway Clearance; Ineffective Thermoregulation; Ineffective Infant Feeding Pattern*

ESSENTIAL DISCHARGE CRITERIA

- Hyperactivity, irritability is controlled
- Takes 90% of prescribed formula
- Mother affirms knowledge that using cocaine while breastfeeding could cause serious injury or death to infant
- Passes no more than three diarrheal stools per day
- Mother participates in care of infant; performs required care techniques
- Parents are knowledgeable about potential problems and appropriate interventions for infants affected by cocaine use during pregnancy
- HIV testing completed for mother and infant per instructional standards
- Referral is made to social and protective services as indicated
- Home environment is verified as safe for infant
- Mother possesses written follow-up appointments
- Parents identify required support services and resources in community

CONGENITAL HEART DEFECT

NURSING DIAGNOSES	OUTCOME CRITERIA	INTERVENTIONS
1 Decreased Cardiac Output *r.t. congenital heart defect, respiratory distress, fluid overload, hypovolemia*	• Maintains VS and BP WNL	• Assess VS qh - auscultate for murmur - provide thermal support • Provide continuous cardiopulmonary monitoring - ensure ECG printer operational • Assess CRT, pulses, skin color q1-4h as indicated • Support infant/family during diagnostic testing - ECG, radiology, echo, cardiac catheterization • Administer digoxin and diuretics as ordered
	• Shows minimal agitation or crying	• Minimize environmental stimulation; provide nesting; offer pacifier; consider analgesics for irritability
		RATIONALE: *C.O. must be supported until palliative or corrective surgery is performed.*
2 Impaired Gas Exchange *r.t. congenital heart defect, pulmonary hypertension, prematurity*	• Maintains oxygenation within parameters for type of congenital heart defect	• Administer O_2 per order - increase flow during feeding • Draw and monitor blood gasses • Provide continuous pulse oximetry and transcutaneous monitoring - pre-, post-ductal as ordered • Feed via gavage if s/s of respiratory distress • Provide comforting strategies, teach to parents
		RATIONALE: *Oxygenation is often compromised due to heart defect. Strategies for improving oxygenation are specific to type of defect, i.e., tetralogy of fallot, septal defect, hypoplastic left heart.*

NURSING DIAGNOSES	OUTCOME CRITERIA	INTERVENTIONS
3 Altered Tissue Perfusion (multisystem) *r.t. decrease in circulating O_2*	• Maintains BP WNL - CRT < 3 sec - pulses not bounding - color pink, no pallor	• Provide continuous hemodynamic monitoring • Administer vasopressor medications as ordered - dopamine • Assess peripheral pulses q2-4h • Assess color, mottling
		RATIONALE: *Strategies to maximize circulation of O_2 to tissues will minimize complications.*
4 Fluid Volume Excess *r.t. cardiac failure*	• Shows no signs of fluid overload - balanced I&O - gains < 20-30 g/day - no edema - breath sounds clear - lab values WNL	• Monitor I&O, perform sp. gr. assessment q2-4h • Restrict fluids, double check fluid administration calculations • Weigh daily, same scale • Administer diuretics as ordered • Auscultate breath sounds bilaterally q2h • Monitor electrolytes • Offer high calorie feedings
		RATIONALE: *Diligent attention to fluid balance will minimize further cardiac compromise.*
5 Nutrition: Less than body requirements *r.t. fatigue, dyspnea, inadequate suck*	• Gains 10-30 g/day	• Weigh daily, same scale • Monitor I&O • Administer TPN, intralipids as ordered
	• Shows no sign of fatigue during feeding	• Offer small, frequent feedings; gavage as indicated - use soft nipple - offer frequent rest periods • Provide continuous cardiac monitoring and/or pulse oximetry during feeding - administer supplemental O_2 as ordered

NURSING DIAGNOSES	OUTCOME CRITERIA	INTERVENTIONS
		• Provide high calorie/low volume feedings
		RATIONALE: *Nutrition essential for growth must be provided in a way to minimize stress and further cardiac compromise.*
6 Activity Intolerance *r.t. cardiac compromise, insufficient oxygenation*	• Tolerates activity with minimal stress	• Feed infant in a sitting-up position • Provide frequent rest periods • Use nipple that causes least stress without overloading suck/swallow • Utilize approach/avoidance behaviors to gauge infant response • Minimize environmental stimulation • Cluster caregiving as infant demonstrates tolerance
		RATIONALE: *The severity of the cardiac defect has a direct effect on activity intolerance.*

OTHER LESS COMMON NURSING DIAGNOSES: *Altered Parenting; Ineffective Feeding Pattern; High Risk for Infection; High Risk for Injury; Inability to Sustain Spontaneous Ventilation; Knowledge Deficit (parents)*

ESSENTIAL DISCHARGE CRITERIA

- Maintains adequate perfusion
- Maintains adequate oxygenation
- Shows no signs of fluid overload
- Tolerates activity with minimal stress
- Parents demonstrate competence with feeding and other complex infant care; such as O_2, medication administration
- Parents verbalize essential nature and plan for follow-up

CONGENITAL HIP DYSPLASIA

NURSING DIAGNOSES	OUTCOME CRITERIA	INTERVENTIONS
1 High Risk for Injury *r.t. delayed identification, treatment of hip dislocation*	• Experiences early detection of dislocation	• Interview parents regarding family tendency for dislocated hips • Perform required inspections for detecting s/s of hip dysplasia - inspect hips for laxity (one or both) - inspect for asymmetry of thigh and gluteal folds - inspect for broadened female perineum (bilateral dislocation) - inspect for Allis's sign (shortened limb on affected side)
	• Has hips abducted whenever checked	• Apply/maintain ordered reduction device depending upon severity of dislocation - preluxation (double diaper, pinning snugly from front to back) - subluxation (Frejka pillow splint with plastic covering) - dislocation (Pavlik harness) - dysplasia (spica cast)
	• Is free of abrasions around cast edges • Shows no cracks in cast	• If casted, place plastic around edges in perineal area; remove, wash plastic each day; watch for cracks, breaks in cast
		RATIONALE: *Facilitate growth of adequate acetabular socket.*
2 High Risk for Impaired Skin Integrity *r.t. irritation, redness, abrasions associated with excretions, irritation from cast edges*	• Displays no coolness, pallor, pulselessness, loss of sensation in lower extremities • CRT WNL	• Inspect, test lower extremities for neurovascular changes q2h - palpate pedal pulses - perform CRT test of nail beds - feel for coolness of legs, feet, toes - inspect for pallor of legs, feet, toes
	• Shows no evidence of tightness, skin abrasions around cast edges - no redness, excoriation, abrasions	• Protect skin - if casted, use foam padding around edges - turn infant q2h; use pillows for supports
		RATIONALE: *Minimize the potential for infection due to broken skin.*

NURSING DIAGNOSES	OUTCOME CRITERIA	INTERVENTIONS
3 Knowledge Deficit *r.t. inexperience with splinting of hip*	• Parents discuss anatomy of dislocation; acknowledge that they will provide consistent follow-up	• Explain anatomy of dislocation - provide diagrams of anatomy of dislocation - remind that treatment is lengthy; consistency is key to success
	• Parents list reportable s/s: absent pedal pulses; pallor, coolness of toes, nailbeds; loss of sensation in feet, toes	• Describe potential complications of splinting; teach assessment, provide list of reportable s/s
	• Parents perform proper care techniques - splinting, diapering, cleansing, cast care - correct feeding techniques: support on pillows at side; if breastfeeding, use football hold - parents possess written follow-up appointments	• Demonstrate required special care; verify follow-up appointments - splint care, diapering, cleansing, skin care - correct feeding, positioning techniques - verify possession of written follow-up appointments
		RATIONALE: *Caregiver understanding of treatment will promote implementation and consistency.*

OTHER LESS COMMON NURSING DIAGNOSES: *Caregiver Role Strain; Ineffective Management of Therapeutic Regimen; Noncompliance*

ESSENTIAL DISCHARGE CRITERIA

- Has clear, intact skin
- Displays no pallor, coolness of feet, toes, nail beds; has intact pedal pulses; CRT of toes, nail beds < 3 sec
- Parents demonstrate correct care techniques: feeding, splinting, cleansing, diapering, positioning, supporting
- Parents possess follow-up appointments

CONGESTIVE HEART FAILURE

NURSING DIAGNOSES	OUTCOME CRITERIA	INTERVENTIONS
1 Decreased Cardiac Output *r.t. pulmonary edema associated with decreased cardiac contractility, structural defect; decreased renal perfusion*	• Serum electrolytes WNL	• Assess serum electrolytes; report deviations
	• Maintains balanced I&O; urinary output 0.5-3 mL/kg/h	• Assess fluid balance • Administer/monitor ordered IV fluids • Administer ordered IV glycoside, diuretic; assess effects • Maintain strict I&O
	• Exhibits no tachycardia, dysrhythmias	• Maintain continuous cardiac monitoring; report deviations • Administer digoxin as ordered
	• Has palpable peripheral pulses, CRT < 3 sec • Shows BP WNL	• Assess peripheral pulses, CRT, and BP q2-4h
	• Displays no pallor, cyanosis; skin warm, dry	• Inspect skin, nail beds, lips, mucous membranes for cyanosis, pallor q2h
		RATIONALE: *Decreased cardiac workload and enhanced cardiac contractility facilitate resolution of disease.*
2 Fluid Volume Excess *r.t. systemic venous engorgement*	• Has decreasing circulating volume; decreasing edema; normalizing electrolytes (K)	• Monitor electrolytes; administer IV fluids and electrolytes as ordered • Assess for edema • Observe QRS complex, waveform for arrhythmia
	• Shows no evidence of distended jugular veins; hepatomegaly; periorbital and facial edema	• Observe for and document - distended neck veins - peripheral or facial edema - hepatomegaly
	• Shows creatinine and BUN WNL • Maintains urinary output 0.5-3 mL/kg/h	• Monitor lab values • Monitor urine output • Administer diuretics as ordered
		RATIONALE: *Controlling fluid volume reduces edema and its effects on healthy tissue.*

NURSING DIAGNOSES	OUTCOME CRITERIA	INTERVENTIONS
3 Impaired Gas Exchange *r.t. pulmonary congestion*	• Shows HR/BP WNL	• Monitor HR and BP q1-2h • Provide continuous cardio-respiratory monitoring
	• Exhibits no signs of pulmonary congestion - no pallor/cyanosis - no tachypnea - no diaphoresis - no hypoxemia - no hypercapnia	• Restrict fluids • Carefully monitor I&O q2h • Administer morphine, diuretics, and vasodilator as ordered • Monitor ABGs and pulse oximetry • Administer O_2 as ordered
	• Exhibits improving respiratory status - RR < 60 breaths per minute - no crackles, moist rales - no pallor, cyanosis; skin warm, dry	• Auscultate chest q1-2h • Assess, foster respiratory sufficiency q2h, per minimum stimulation protocol - assess RR - auscultate breath sounds - inspect skin, nail beds, lips, mucous membranes for cyanosis, pallor - elevate head, chest
		RATIONALE: *Adequate gas exchange must be maintained to prevent tissue damage to other organ systems. Reducing circulating fluids decreases pulmonary fluid overload.*
4 Altered Nutrition: Less than body requirements *r.t. anorexia, dyspnea, fatigue, poor feeding*	• Body weight WNL or normalizing	• Weigh daily, naked, same scale
	• Takes 80% or more of feedings	• Maintain required nutrition - give frequent, small feedings; use higher formula concentration (24 cal/oz) to maintain calorie intake without excessive fluids, per orders - increase size of nipple hole to decrease sucking efforts - blow O_2 around face area while feeding, if needed to reduce exertional dyspnea
		RATIONALE: *Increased work of breathing is associated with CHF, which decreases the infant's energy reserve and ability to taking feedings and/or maximize calorie intake.*

NURSING DIAGNOSES	OUTCOME CRITERIA	INTERVENTIONS
5 High Risk for Injury (cardiac complications) *r.t. digoxin toxicity*	• Shows no arrhythmias; no ECG changes	• Monitor apical pulse: rate, rhythm continuously per ECG monitor
	• Apical pulse is 110-160 bpm	• Withhold digoxin if PR interval > 0.16 sec, HR irregular, or if bradycardia (< 90 bpm); notify physician • Double check digoxin with nurse before administering
	• Serum K WNL	• Withhold digoxin if serum K below required level; notify physician
	• Heart sounds are free of gallop, murmur, rub	• Assess heart sounds for evidence of: gallop, murmur, rub; notify physician
		RATIONALE: *The narrow range between therapeutic and toxic levels places the preterm infant at increased risk for toxicity.*
6 High Risk for Fluid Volume Deficit *r.t. diuretic medication*	• Maintains balanced I&O; takes required fluids	• Double check diuretic meds with nurse before administration • Monitor, maintain balanced I&O q4h - administer ordered oral, parenteral fluids
	• Shows good skin turgor, moist mucous membranes	• Assess skin turgor, mucous membranes q4-8h
	• Shows serum (Na and K), electrolytes, BUN, creative blood gases WNL	• Monitor electrolytes, blood gases qd
		RATIONALE: *Diuretic therapy places the infant at risk due to the immaturity of the kidney and other circulatory problems.*

NURSING DIAGNOSES	OUTCOME CRITERIA	INTERVENTIONS
7 Knowledge Deficit *r.t. infant's illness, prognosis, hospitalization, complex home care*	• Parents discuss physiology of CHF; ask appropriate questions	• Explain pathophysiology of CHF; provide written information
	• Parents list ways to prevent stressful factors for infant; demonstrate energy conserving strategies	• Discuss methods of energy conservation: anticipate hunger, keep dry, comfortable; hold, cuddle, rock, respond to infant signals
	• Parents successfully feed, hold, soothe infant	• Demonstrate feeding, holding, soothing, positioning
	• Parents describe reportable s/s of impending CHF: dyspnea, anorexia, rapid pulse, irregular pulse	• Describe, provide list of reportable s/s
	• Parents discuss medications: effects, side effects, dosage	• Discuss, explain medications and their relationship to s/s; review medications: effects, side effects, dosages
	• Parents verbalize confidence in ability to manage home care - parents identify community support persons/group - parents identify source of emergency care - parents possess written follow-up appointments	• Facilitate planning for home care - make appropriate referrals to community health resources, support groups, financial services, social services - provide phone numbers for emergency care, physician - verify written appointments for follow-up care

RATIONALE: *Knowledgeable, competent parents are likely to provide safe, uncomplicated home care.*

OTHER LESS COMMON NURSING DIAGNOSES: *Ineffective Breathing Pattern; High Risk for Infection; Altered Growth and Development; Ineffective Infant Feeding Pattern; High Risk for Altered Parenting*

ESSENTIAL DISCHARGE CRITERIA

- Maintains balanced I&O; has no edema
- Shows normal serum electrolytes
- Has clear breath sounds; no respiratory distress
- Body weight is normalizing
- Shows no cardiac arrhythmias; no ECG changes
- Parents demonstrate ability to manage C.O.-related care at home, including appropriate assessments and safe medications administration
- Parents demonstrate effective feeding techniques
- Parents express understanding of long-term health management goals
- Parents have list of reportable s/s and written follow-up appointment

FEEDING DYSFUNCTION

NURSING DIAGNOSES	OUTCOME CRITERIA	INTERVENTIONS
1 Ineffective Infant Feeding Pattern *r.t. inability to begin or maintain effective coordination of sucking, swallowing, and breathing*	• Receives adequate nutrition for age/need, appropriate for growth	• Assess feeding ability as it relates to gestational age - non-nutritive suck - nutritive suck - suck/swallow/rest pattern - oxygenation/respiratory effort during feedings • Collaborate with dietitian/ physician/feeding specialist to set goals for caloric intake needed for weight gain
	• Shows increasing skill in oral intake (for developmental level)	• Provide infant with specific opportunities that promote effective oral feedings based on assessment and plan for caloric intake - encourage non-nutritive sucking - set pattern for feeding/sleep/wake cycle - provide quiet, restful area for feeding, i.e., dim lights, reduce noise/activity - provide appropriate nipple for ability - contain infant securely in blanket and caregiver arms - use neutral head positioning, both hands in midline close to face, avoid face-to-face contact between infant and caregiver (too stimulating) - assess whether rocking during suck/swallow phase is too stimulating - support tongue and cheeks during suck/swallow cycle if necessary - burp infant approximately every 15-20 mL, using a gentle pat or massage on infant's back
		RATIONALE: *Prematurity and/or neurologic impairment affects suck/swallow/breath coordination. Interventions to support the neonate's integration of feeding skills will facilitate efficient use of calories and minimize complications, i.e., aspiration.*

NURSING DIAGNOSES	OUTCOME CRITERIA	INTERVENTIONS
2 High Risk for Altered Parenting *r.t. feelings of inadequacy in ability to feed infant*	• Parents demonstrate increased skill in feeding	• Involve parents in determining which interventions are most effective in increasing oral intake - plan to spend time with parents when they feed infant - provide encouragement, guidance, and feedback - demonstrate techniques as needed, but support parent skill acquisition as first priority
	• Parents actively involve selves in all feeding activities	• Involve parents in determining goals for discharge based on feeding ability, caloric intake, weight gain • Provide referrals to community agencies for support after discharge
		RATIONALE: *Knowledgeable, competent parents are likely to succeed in achieving and maintaining the infant's required nutrition.*

OTHER LESS COMMON NURSING DIAGNOSES:

Altered Nutrition: Less than body requirements; Fluid Volume deficit

ESSENTIAL DISCHARGE CRITERIA

- Shows steady pattern of weight gain based on appropriate caloric intake
- Parents demonstrate consistent ability to meet caloric intake for infant through mutually agreed-upon methods of feeding
- Parents verbalize plan for follow-up and weight checks

FETAL ALCOHOL SYNDROME

NURSING DIAGNOSES	OUTCOME CRITERIA	INTERVENTIONS
1 Sleep Pattern Disturbance *r.t. alcohol, withdrawal symptoms*	• Demonstrates normal sleep pattern between feedings, i.e., quiet sleep - sleeps for 20-30 min periods	• Swaddle infant, place side-lying or prone • Provide quiet area with dimmed lighting during sleep periods • Provide feedings on a regular basis
	• Responds to soothing, cuddling, holding	• Provide vertical rocking to quiet • Provide non-nutritive sucking • Involve parents in soothing infant • Consider use of "cuddlers" or "foster grandparents" to provide extended periods of holding/rocking infant during acute phase
		RATIONALE: *Establishment of regular sleep pattern promotes adequate growth and development during newborn period.*
2 Potential for Injury *r.t. seizures, drug withdrawals*	• Demonstrates no signs of withdrawal - no irritability - no high pitched, shrill cry - no hyperactivity, tumors - no seizures	• Observe for signs of seizure activity; report as indicated - lip smacking - jitteriness vs. seizure - blinking eyes - nystagmus • Provide soothing, cuddling, holding (see above) • Administer medications as ordered - paregoric - phenobarbital - valium
		RATIONALE: *Withdrawal may be demonstrated by a range of behaviors from tremors to irritability to clonic seizure. Interventions focus on assessment and timely intervention.*

NURSING DIAGNOSES	OUTCOME CRITERIA	INTERVENTIONS
3 High Risk for Fluid Volume Deficit *r.t. diarrhea associated with bowel hypermotility and altered fluid intake*	• Maintains balanced I&O	• Maintain strict I&O; administer ordered parenteral fluids
	• Urinary output and sp. gr. WNL	• Weigh diapers • Assess urine sp. gr. q4h
	• Serum K WNL	• Monitor serum K; report deviations
	• Has moist mucous membranes, good skin turgor	• Inspect mucous membranes, skin q4h
	• Fontanels are not depressed	• Inspect fontanels q4h
	• Shows no weight loss	• Weigh daily or as ordered
	• Has decreasing number of diarrhea, stools per day	• Monitor, record stools: amount, character, frequency
		RATIONALE: *GI distress may lead to inadequate calorie consumption for growth.*
4 Altered Nutrition: Less than body requirements *r.t. maternal malnutrition, infant gastrointestinal irritability, excess catabolism*	• Demonstrates adequate nutrition - body weight stable or increasing - balanced I&O - serum glucose and electrolytes WNL	• Assess nutritional intake - weigh daily - maintain I&O - monitor serum glucose and electrolytes
	• Takes, retains 100-200 cal/kg/day without abdominal distention	• Maintain intake, retention of nutrition - offer small, frequent feeds (start with half-strength formula) - position on side post feed; observe for uncoordinated sucking, swallowing, regurgitation gavage as needed - consider concentrated formula of 24 cal/oz if no weight gain - maintain patent IV line for unstable infant
	• Mother demonstrates required skill in feeding infant - acknowledges inappropriate breastfeeding situations	• Involve mother in providing feeding - discuss breastfeeding restrictions • Teach quieting strategies

NURSING DIAGNOSES	OUTCOME CRITERIA	INTERVENTIONS
		RATIONALE: *FAS infants usually have IUGR requiring increased calories for growth.*
5 Impaired Skin Integrity *r.t. diarrhea stools, hyperactivity*	• Perianal skin is clear, intact	• Protect perianal area - gently cleanse perianal area after each stool - apply location, oil - expose excoriated perianal area to air at frequent intervals
	• Knees, elbows, face are free of redness, irritation	• Protect from scratches, sheet burns - pad elbows, knees - place sheepskin under face - apply mittens to prevent scratching - provide waterbed mattress
		RATIONALE: *The side effects of irritability and GI distress increase the risk for skin breakdown.*
6 Altered Parenting *r.t. unstable family, alcohol abuse by mother*	• Mother makes positive comments about self, infant	• Allow time for mother to discuss feelings about self, infant
	• Mother holds, cuddles, talks to infant; initiates, desires contact with infant; demonstrates required care skills	• Encourage mother/infant contact - encourage mother to hold, cuddle, soothe infant - demonstrate care techniques as required - listen to maternal fears about infant care skills
	• Mother participates in discussion of need for alcohol rehabilitation; identifies support groups, persons	• Discuss mother's need for, willingness to participate in alcohol rehabilitation program
	• Infant responds to holding, cuddling, soothing behaviors	• Identify if infant is unresponsive to mothering; refer mother to professional child care counseling to learn coping skills
	• Infant is discharged to home verified as safe	• Refer to social or protective services for home evaluation

NURSING DIAGNOSES	OUTCOME CRITERIA	INTERVENTIONS
		RATIONALE: *Addiction may interfere with the mother's ability to care for the infant. The patient will require support and counseling with intensive follow-up, which often includes mandatory reporting.*
7 Knowledge Deficit *r.t. mother's care of infant at home*	• Expresses feelings about infant care; performs bathing, dressing, feeding, medicating, holding, cuddling, stimulation	• Facilitate home care planning - schedule time for listening, teaching - demonstrate infant care techniques - explain medication administration - discuss need to remain drug free; that breast milk transmits drugs, alcohol
	• Describes s/s of infant alcohol withdrawal (see ND #2)	• Review, provide list of s/s of infant alcohol withdrawal
	• Identifies support groups/persons; potential need for foster care	• Discuss needed lifestyle changes; need for support; potential need for foster care
		RATIONALE: *Knowledgeable, competent parents are more likely to provide timely, appropriate care.*

OTHER LESS COMMON NURSING DIAGNOSES: *Altered Growth and Development; Hyperthermia; High Risk for Infection; Diarrhea; Altered Family Process*

ESSENTIAL DISCHARGE CRITERIA

- Hyperactivity, irritability is controlled
- Takes, retains 90% of prescribed formula with demonstrated weight gain
- Passes no more than three diarrheal stools per day
- Mother participates in care of infant; performs required care techniques
- Mother discusses need for drug rehabilitation, lifestyle changes
- Mother identifies support groups/persons
- Home environment is verified as safe for infant
- Mother has realistic plans for complying with follow-up requirements
- Referral is made to social and protective services as indicated

GASTROSCHISIS/OMPHALOCELE

NURSING DIAGNOSES	OUTCOME CRITERIA	INTERVENTIONS
1 High Risk for Injury *r.t. exposure of intestinal contents, compromised circulation to the defect* *(Refer to "Pre-op" and "Post-op" care plans)*	• Exposed intestines are pink, warm; sac remains intact until surgery	• Apply warm, sterile normal saline-soaked gauze to defect - cover with plastic wrap • Support defect to minimize twisting, crimping of defect - suspend as ordered
	• Shows soft, flat abdomen	• Assess abdomen for firmness, tenderness, redness, loops of bowel • Note x-ray results • Place NG/OG tube; leave open to air or low intermittent suction as ordered
		RATIONALE: *It is essential to maintain good blood supply to the defect to minimize necrosis prior to surgical repair.*
2 High Risk for Infection *r.t. abdominal wall defect, depressed immune response, surgical intervention*	• Shows VS WNL • Abdominal incision dry, intact, no drainage	• Assess VS q2h, report as indicated • Administer antibiotics as ordered • Utilize universal precautions • Assess incision q2-4h - apply antimicrobial ointment as ordered • Change dressing per unit standard
		RATIONALE: *Infants have a sluggish immune response and incomplete antibody coverage.*
3 Ineffective Thermo-regulation *r.t. abdominal defect, increased surface area, presence of moist compress*	• Shows temperature WNL - extremities warm - no mottling	• Assess temperature q1-2h • Initiate servo control mechanism in isolette or open warmer • Ensure presence of warm N/S soaks to defect prior to surgery • Minimize drafts
		RATIONALE: *The abdominal defect increases the infant's surface area, enabling increase heat loss.*

NURSING DIAGNOSES	OUTCOME CRITERIA	INTERVENTIONS
4 Nutrition: Less than body requirements *r.t. NPO status, feeding intolerance, increased calorie requirements*	• Shows consistent weight gain	• Weigh daily, naked, on the same scale - report loss/gain > 30 g • Administer IV fluids, TPN, intralipids as ordered • Assess IV sites hourly, change site as soon as infiltration noted
	• Takes, retains 90% of feeding • Has no vomiting	• Encourage non-nutritive sucking • Initiates oral feedings as ordered (see "Gastrostomy" care plan) - continuous feedings - high calorie formula - small, frequent feedings
		RATIONALE: *Maintenance of IV access is essential to ensure adequate fluid/nutrition intake until adequate enteral feeding can be established.*
5 Ineffective Breathing Pattern *r.t. pressure from abdominal contents (post-op)*	• Establishes a normal, effective breathing pattern	• Assess respiratory status qh • Provide continuous cardiopulmonary monitoring • Discuss reduction of intestines into abdomen with surgeon • Anticipate need for O_2 and suction
		RATIONALE: *Reduction of intestines into abdomen may increase pressure on the diaphragm to the point of respiratory compromise.*
6 Altered Parenting *r.t. separation at birth, surgical intervention*	• See "Pre-op" and "Post-op" care plans	

COMP NEONATE

NURSING DIAGNOSES	OUTCOME CRITERIA	INTERVENTIONS
7 Knowledge Deficit *r.t. lack of experience with problem*	• See "Pre-op" and "Post-op" care plans	

OTHER LESS COMMON NURSING DIAGNOSES: *High Risk for Fluid Volume Deficit; Pain; Impaired Skin Integrity*

ESSENTIAL DISCHARGE CRITERIA

- Takes, retains 90% of feedings
- Gains weight daily
- Incision well healed, no drainage or redness
- Parents demonstrate competence with feeding method
- Parents possess written instructions and follow-up appointments
- Parents identify community resources, as indicated

GASTROSTOMY

NURSING DIAGNOSES	OUTCOME CRITERIA	INTERVENTIONS
1 High Risk for Impaired Skin Integrity *r.t. moist skin, surgical site*	• Shows dry, intact skin at gastrostomy site	• Provide gastrostomy site care q8-24h - cleanse with half-strength H_2O_2 • Place gauze dressing at site prn
		RATIONALE: *The moist stoma and administration of feedings provide a source for skin breakdown and/or infection.*
2 High Risk for Injury *r.t. tube displacement, clogged tube*	• Has intact gastrostomy tube in proper location	• Stabilize gastrostomy tube with slit nipple • Bundle infant to minimize grasping of tube • Apply mittens as indicated • Mark tube to provide easy visualization of proper placement • Flush tube with sterile water after feeding
		RATIONALE: *As the infant recovers and his/her activity increases, the potential for tube dislodgment increases.*
3 Knowledge Deficit *r.t. gastrostomy care and/or feeding*	• Parents demonstrate gastrostomy care	• Demonstrate gastrostomy care - provide handouts - provide site care - provide dislodgment plan
	• Parents demonstrate care and feeding of infant	• Discuss feeding plan, provide handouts • Teach gastrostomy feeding technique • Demonstrate oral feedings and/or stimulation as appropriate
	• Parents verbalize sources for equipment needs	• Refer to local vendors for gastrostomy care equipment • Consult social work • Assist parents in developing plan for placement of supplies in home, when to restock

NURSING DIAGNOSES	OUTCOME CRITERIA	INTERVENTIONS
		RATIONALE: *Parents that are knowledgeable and demonstrate competency will have increased chance of success.*

OTHER LESS COMMON NURSING DIAGNOSES: *Ineffective Infant Feeding Pattern; Ineffective Airway Clearance; Pain; Altered Nutrition: Less than body requirements*

ESSENTIAL DISCHARGE CRITERIA

- Takes, retains 90% of feedings
- Gains weight daily
- Parents demonstrate skill with feeding techniques
- Parents identify home care plan, supply source, community resources
- Parents possess printed information regarding care
- Parents verbalize importance of care, and have follow-up appointments

NURSING DIAGNOSES	OUTCOME CRITERIA	INTERVENTIONS
1 High Risk for Infection *r.t. inadequate secondary defenses; immunodeficiency*	• Is free of s/s of infection - VS WNL - normal appetite - color appropriate for race	• Assess for s/s of infection - fever - increased pulse and respirations - pallor - lethargy • Monitor VS q4h • Administer antibiotics, antiviral and antifungal medications as ordered • Administer IVIG as ordered
	• Experiences no cough or rhinorrhea	• Use aseptic technique with invasive procedures • Assess for cough, nasal congestion, and adventitious breath sounds q8h • Provide pulmonary hygiene - turn frequently - apply gentle oral suction if needed
	• Shows WBC count with differential WNL	• Monitor CBC with differential - watch for neutropenia
	• Displays intact skin without rashes, abrasions	• Assess skin qd for rash, lesions, drainage • Provide proper hygiene - keep skin clean, dry, and well lubricated
	• Shows no nosocomial infections	• Maintain universal precautions; explain precautions to family/visitors • Instruct all visitors to wash hands before and after entering the patient's room • Wash hands before and after caring for the patient to prevent cross-contamination of patients • Wear gloves for all patient contacts • Wear mask and protective eye wear if aeration or splattering is likely to occur • Place used needles and syringes immediately in an impermeable container; do not recap needles

NURSING DIAGNOSES	OUTCOME CRITERIA	INTERVENTIONS
		RATIONALE: *Early detection and prompt treatment decrease progress of infection. Meticulous compliance with infection control measures protects child from nosocomial and other infections.*
2 Altered Protection *r.t. immunodeficiency*	• Experiences prompt treatment of bacterial and treatable opportunistic infections	• Assess for s/s of possible infection q1-4h
	• Is free of toxic side effects (macrocytosis, anemia, neutropenia) if antiretroviral agents are administered	• Monitor Hct, Hb, WBC count, cell differential while on antiretroviral therapy
	• Demonstrates adequate nutritional intake - normal weight gain - takes, retains feedings	• Weigh daily; assess type and amount of dietary intake; ensure adequate calories daily
		RATIONALE: *Prompt identification of infection, adequate nutrition, and possible use of antiretroviral agents may lessen progress of this disease in neonates.*
3 Interrupted Breastfeeding *r.t. possibility that HIV virus may be transmitted through human milk*	• Mother demonstrates knowledge that breastfeeding is not recommended	• Discuss with the mother the theories related to HIV transmission during the breastfeeding process (that breastfeeding is not recommended due to other feeding options available) • Provide emotional support
		RATIONALE: *The risk of HIV infection transmission to infants born to seropositive mothers can be reduced to approximately 20% when breastfeeding is not chosen as mode of infant feeding.*

NURSING DIAGNOSES	OUTCOME CRITERIA	INTERVENTIONS
4 High Risk for Altered Parenting *r.t. maternal and/or infant diagnosis of AIDS*	• Parents demonstrate knowledge of possible disease process, course, and care of infant with this possible diagnosis - acknowledge awareness of incidence of infection in additional pregnancies	• Counsel and educate parents regarding - possible course of disease process - how disease is transmitted - infant care - incidence of infection in subsequent pregnancies • Provide emotional support **RATIONALE:** *Parents will be more confident caring for infant if they are well informed concerning the disease process, its course, and infant care.*
5 High Risk for Caregiver Role Strain *r.t. instability of caregiver's health*	• Parents demonstrate knowledge of normal baby care and special care of infant with possible HIV diagnosis	• Explain to parents and other caregivers: normal baby care, universal precautions **RATIONALE:** *Due to possible instability of mother's health, other caregivers should be taught to care for infant when the mother is not able or needs a break.*

OTHER LESS COMMON NURSING DIAGNOSES: *Ineffective Family Coping: Compromised; Knowledge Deficit; Altered Growth and Development*

ESSENTIAL DISCHARGE CRITERIA

- Is free of symptoms of infection
- Maintains adequate nutrition
- Is free of side effects of AZT therapy
- Parents verbalize knowledge of disease process and infant care
- Parents possess follow-up appointments, list of community resources

HYDROCEPHALUS

NURSING DIAGNOSES	OUTCOME CRITERIA	INTERVENTIONS

See "Preoperative Care" and "Postoperative Care" care plans

NURSING DIAGNOSES	OUTCOME CRITERIA	INTERVENTIONS
1 High Risk for Impaired Skin Integrity *r.t. pressure, shape, and weight of the head*	• Has intact skin; no redness or broken areas	• Assess head for signs of skin breakdown q4h • Change and support head position q2h • Use waterbed/pillow • Keep skin clean and dry • Do not position head on shunt side immediately post-operatively **RATIONALE:** *Prevention of pressure sores is essential because of immobility.*
2 High Risk for Altered Parenting *r.t. interruption of bonding process, lack of acceptance of condition, lack of knowledge*	• Parents demonstrate bonding/attachment behavior - visits and/or calls regularly - desires to participate in caregiving activities - verbalizes comfort in ability to care for infant	• Assess learning needs of patient • Teach parents how to care for infant and observe them giving care; involve them in infant's care as much as possible • Provide information about additional supportive resources • Normalize care as much as possible **RATIONALE:** *Knowledge and skill combine to reduce parent anxiety and provide sense of support.*
3 Sensory/ Perceptual Alterations *r.t. increasing intracranial pressure*	• Experiences prompt reversal of any s/s of increasing intracranial pressure - fontanel tension - head circumference - scalp vein distension - feeding, vomiting - altered LOC	• Assess for signs of increased intracranial pressure q8h - anterior fontanel tense, full, or bulging - accelerated head growth - scalp thin and shiny - scalp vein distention - vomiting, poor feeding - irritability - seizures • Elevate HOB • Measure head circumference daily

NURSING DIAGNOSES	OUTCOME CRITERIA	INTERVENTIONS
		• Organize care to decrease fatigue • Minimize noxious stimuli (decrease noise, dim lights, minimize handling)
		RATIONALE: *Early detection and prompt management of neurologic function and status is essential to prevent cerebral hypoxia.*

OTHER LESS COMMON NURSING DIAGNOSES: *Altered Tissue Perfusion (intracranial); Pain; Altered Nutrition: Less than body requirements; Caregiver Role Strain; Ineffective Thermoregulation; Ineffective Breathing Pattern*

ESSENTIAL DISCHARGE CRITERIA

- Shows intact or healing skin
- Has no signs of increased intracranial pressure
- Parents demonstrate ability to care for infant
- Parents verbalize understanding of resources available and the importance of follow-up

HYPERBILIRUBINEMIA

NURSING DIAGNOSES	OUTCOME CRITERIA	INTERVENTIONS
1 High Risk for Injury *r.t. mental retardation, death associated with increased bilirubin levels*	• Shows no evidence of s/s of hyperbilirubinemia - jaundice - delayed stools - dark, concentrated urine - lethargy - poor feeding - absent Moro reflex - high pitched cry - tremors, irritability, seizures	• Identify risk factors - bruising - sepsis - delayed cord clamping - mother with diabetes - SGA - plethora - Rh, ABO incompatibility • Assess newborn for s/s of hyperbilirubinemia on admission and q2-4h first 5 days of life • Assess for s/s of hyperbilirubinemia q2-4h; report s/s
	• Shows serum bilirubin WNL for age	• Monitor bilirubin levels; report increases outside parameters
	• Hb, Hct stable, normal	• Monitor Hb and Hct; report decreases
	• Shows no increase in reticulocytes	• Monitor reticulocytes; report increases
	• Shows bilirubin levels decreasing after 2-3 days	• Provide phototherapy - follow protocols for timing, duration, procedure - monitor bilirubin level q6-12h while under therapy
	• Maintains VS within safe limits during and after exchange	• Prepare for ordered exchange transfusion - monitor VS during and after transfusion; report deviations - verify blood out/blood in per unit standard

RATIONALE: *Elevated bilirubin levels can cross the blood-brain barrier and cause straining of the brain and neurologic sequelae.*

NURSING DIAGNOSES	OUTCOME CRITERIA	INTERVENTIONS
2 High Risk for Fluid Volume Deficit *r.t. phototherapy*	• Loses less than 10% of body weight; takes prescribed amounts of feedings	• Maintain fluid intake - continue prescribed feeding schedule - weigh qd - maintain I&O - provide extra oral or IV fluids if excess weight loss, elevated temperature, loose stools, concentrated urine per physician's order
	• Shows urine output of 2-3 mL/kg/h - urine color becomes less dark, concentrated - soft, not liquid stools	• Assess output - monitor color, amount of urine q1-4h - monitor stools for looseness q1-4h
	• Maintains fluid balance - body temperature WNL - moist mucous membranes; fontanels not depressed	• Assess hydration - monitor body temperature q2h if on constant monitor, q3-4h with feedings if done manually - inspect mucous membranes, fontanels
		RATIONALE: *Exposure to phototherapy is an additional source of insensible water loss.*
3 Impaired Skin Integrity *r.t. effect of phototherapy*	• Displays no evidence of conjunctivitis	• Place eye patches on infant during therapy; remove at least q4h to inspect eyes
	• Displays no macropapular rash	• Inspect skin q4h; report rash
	• Shows no skin irritation of genitals or perianal region	• Shield genitals during therapy; keep diaper area clean, dry to reduce irritation - apply water-base ointment to excoriated areas as ordered
		RATIONALE: *Phototherapy has common side effects of dry skin, rash, eye irritation, diarrheal stools.*

NURSING DIAGNOSES	OUTCOME CRITERIA	INTERVENTIONS
4 High Risk of Injury *r.t. life threatening side effects associated with exchange transfusion*	• Has bilirubin, Hb, Hct performed on blood draw with minimal exposure to fluorescent light	• Monitor pre- and post-transfusion levels of bilirubin, Hb, Hct, other tests as ordered
	• Shows post-transfusion bilirubin level no more than half of pre-transfusion level	• Monitor bilirubin q4-6h x 24h post transfusion, then 8-12h as indicated
	• Maintains BP, HR; temperature WNL, for size, during and after procedure	• Electronically monitor - BP and HR q10 min during exchange procedure; q15-30 min after procedure for 2 h then routine schedule - axillary temperature q30 min (provide radiant heater)
	• Shows no evidence of aspiration during transfusion	• Aspirate stomach before procedure - leave OG tube open to air
	• Experiences prompt treatment of cardiac arrest, other critical events	• Keep resuscitation equipment at bedside; administer parenteral fluids per orders
	• Displays no evidence of intestinal perforation post-transfusion - bloody stools - abdominal distention - hypotension - cyanosis - bloody OG aspirant - vomiting	• Assess for s/s of intestinal perforation q2-24h - abdominal skin color, tension - loops of bowel - test stool for blood - inspect OG aspirant
	• Takes required nutrition, fluids post-transfusion	• Resume feedings, oral or nasogastric, post-transfusion to maintain caloric, fluid requirements per unit standards - anticipate NPO status for 12-24h

RATIONALE: *Exchange transfusion is instituted to protect the CNS status. The removal and introduction of fresh blood places the infant at risk for cardiovascular and/or intravascular compromise.*

NURSING DIAGNOSES	OUTCOME CRITERIA	INTERVENTIONS
5 High Risk for Altered Parenting *r.t. separation, interrupted bonding*	• Parents feed, hold, touch, diaper, talk to infant	• Maintain parental contact - remove from phototherapy for mother's visit as indicated - encourage parents to feed, hold, diaper infant
	• Parents verbalize feelings, concerns	• Take time to listen to parents' fears, concerns
		RATIONALE: *Parents alter their birth plans to incorporate the unexpected need for intervention.*
6 Knowledge Deficit *r.t. condition of infant, care of child at home*	• Parents discuss physiology of condition, treatment rationale	• Provide factual information about physiology of illness - answer questions - clarify misconceptions - provide literature about hyperbilirubinemia
	• Parents ask appropriate questions	• Be alert to inappropriate questions that signal misunderstanding
	• Parents participate in feeding, diapering, holding	• Involve parents in care to maximize skills, confidence with care at home
	• Parents list reportable s/s: jaundice in 5-7 days, elevated temperature, lethargy, rigidity of muscles, irritability, high pitched cry, seizures, poor feeding	• Discuss reportable s/s; significance of each symptom
	• Parents possess written follow-up appointments	• Verify possession of follow-up appointments
		RATIONALE: *Although physiologic jaundice is fairly common, hyperbilirubinemia requiring intervention and/or exchange necessitates directed parent education.*

OTHER LESS COMMON NURSING DIAGNOSES: *Ineffective Feeding Pattern; Altered Nutrition; Diarrhea; Fluid Volume Excess; Altered Tissue Perfusion (GI)*

ESSENTIAL DISCHARGE CRITERIA

- Serum bilirubin decreasing; Hct, Hb, reticulocytes, platelets normalizing
- Takes, retains at least 90% of prescribed feedings
- Maintains balanced I&O
- Shows no abdominal distention
- Shows urine of normal color: clear, amber
- Lusty cry, not high pitched
- Parents demonstrate safe, effective care techniques
- Parents list reportable s/s, possess follow-up phone numbers

HYPOCALCEMIA

NURSING DIAGNOSES	OUTCOME CRITERIA	INTERVENTIONS
1 High Risk for Injury (internal) *r.t. respiratory distress, seizures, death associated with hypocalcemia*	• Shows no s/s of symptomatic hypocalcemia - tremors - muscle twitching - irritability - poor feeding - hypoglycemia	• Assess infant on admission for high risk factors - prematurity - asphyxia - mother with diabetes - renal disease - medications: bicarbonate, furosemide, citrate blood • Assess high risk infants for s/s of hypocalcemia and hypoglycemia; report as indicated and initiate prompt treatment
	• Shows serum Ca and phosphorus levels WNL	• Assess Ca, phosphorus levels; report low levels; initiate prompt treatment per orders
	• Displays no seizure activity	• Protect high risk infant - minimize movement, handling of infant - maintain calm, quiet environment
	• Maintain HR > 100 bpm during Ca gluconate infusion	• Prepare, administer ordered Ca gluconate infusion following agency protocol - monitor HR, pulse using continuous cardiac monitoring during infusions - report bradycardia; stop infusion - report, stop infusion if vomiting
	• Maintains Ca:PO_4 at 4:6	• Monitor Ca:PO_4 ratio
	• Parents list reportable s/s	• Describe reportable s/s: tremors, twitching; discuss significance

RATIONALE: *Hypocalcemia is often asymptomatic with asphyxia, IDM, VLBW infants necessitating attentiveness to observation.*

NURSING DIAGNOSES	OUTCOME CRITERIA	INTERVENTIONS
2 Impaired Tissue Integrity *r.t. chemical irritants associated with infusions*	• Displays no evidence of redness, swelling around infusion site during transfusion - no tissue necrosis, extravasation post-infusions	• Monitor infusion - carefully inspect infusion site; discontinue and apply pressure to site for 1 min if any evidence of redness, swelling - inspect line for patency - inspect line for evidence of precipitate; if present, stop infusion • Administer Wydase as ordered for infiltration
		RATIONALE: *Ca infusions can cause chemical burns and skin slough when infiltrated.*
3 Knowledge Deficit *r.t. lack of experience in use of Ca supplements and monitoring of child at home*	• Parents discuss physiology of condition, treatment rationale; ask appropriate questions	• Teach physiology of condition; encourage questions, discussion
	• Parents discuss need to minimize handling, stimulation until condition stabilizes	• Review and demonstrate care techniques - limited handling - limited stimulation until stabilized
	• Parents perform formula preparation - name of Ca supplement - correct measurement - correct addition to formula - name of formula - tapering of dosage	• Demonstrate, explain how to add Ca medication, need to taper Ca supplements per orders to prevent rebound hypocalcemia
	• Parents list reportable s/s: irritability, twitching, tonic posturing, incoordinated eye or mouth movements	• Describe reportable s/s and reasons for significance
	• Parents possess written follow-up appointments	• Verify possession of follow-up appointments
		RATIONALE: *Although rare, the need for home Ca therapy requires careful attention to dosage and symptom assessment.*

OTHER LESS COMMON NURSING DIAGNOSES: *Ineffective Infant Feeding Pattern; Diarrhea; High Risk for Altered Parenting*

ESSENTIAL DISCHARGE CRITERIA

- Shows no s/s of symptomatic hypocalcemia
- Parents discuss physiology of condition
- Parents perform formula preparation with Ca supplement
- Parents list reportable s/s and possess written follow-up appointments

HYPOGLYCEMIA

NURSING DIAGNOSES	OUTCOME CRITERIA	INTERVENTIONS
1 Altered Nutrition: Less than body requirements *r.t. lack of circulating glucose*	• Shows glucose levels WNL	• Monitor glucose levels per unit standard
	• Takes oral fluids sufficient to maintain glucose levels	• Assess type and amount of PO dietary intake • Give IV fluids as ordered • Monitor I&O
	• Maintains normal glucose levels with IV therapy	• If oral fluids inadequate to maintain normal glucose levels, institute IV therapy, per orders
	• Shows no s/s of hypoglycemia	• Assess for s/s of hypoglycemia, including tremors, jitteriness, abnormal cry, apnea, irregular respirations, cyanosis, lethargy, hypotonia, seizure activity
		RATIONALE: *Glucose is an essential energy source for growth and development.*
2 High Risk for Altered Body Temperature *r.t. cold stress, prematurity*	• Maintains stable body temperature	• Assess temperature q2h • Use a thermal-neutral environment to maintain body temperature WNL
		RATIONALE: *Cold stress causes rapid depletion of glycogen.*
3 Ineffective Breathing Patterns *r.t. hypoglycemia*	• Is free of respiratory distress	• Assess RR, rhythm, and depth q1-3h • Assess infant for signs of respiratory distress including grunting, flaring, retracting
		RATIONALE: *Respiratory distress results in increased energy use and thus increased utilization of glucose and the potential for lactic acidosis.*

NURSING DIAGNOSES	OUTCOME CRITERIA	INTERVENTIONS
4 Altered Protection *r.t. conditions identified that predispose infants to hypoglycemia*	• Experiences early detection of high risk factors - preterm infant - SGA infant - LGA infant - IDM	• Assess gestational age of infant on admission • Assess body weight, length, and head circumference to determine if size is appropriate for gestational age
		RATIONALE: *Early detection of predisposition to hypoglycemia leads to prompt prevention and management measures.*
5 Knowledge Deficit *r.t. interruption in bonding process, lack of experience*	• Parents maintain frequent contact with infant • Parents verbalize knowledge of infant's disease process	• Encourage parents to visit often; engage them in caring for their infant as much as possible
	• Parents verbalize knowledge of infant care	• Educate parents in normal infant care in preparation for discharge
		RATIONALE: *Parents gain confidence in parenting when encouraged to participate in infant's care and when knowledgeable about what is happening to their infant.*
6 Interrupted Breastfeeding *r.t. infant illness* *(Refer to "Breastfeeding" care plan)*	• Mother maintains milk supply	• Review with mother - techniques to pump breasts manually or with an electric breast pump - pumping frequency - fluid and nutrition needs
	• Mother resumes breastfeeding as soon as infant is physically able	• Educate and support mother in breastfeeding techniques • Provide written materials and community resources
		RATIONALE: *Mothers may provide breast milk for their infants. Mothers who are educated and supported in the breastfeeding process will breastfeed longer.*

OTHER LESS COMMON NURSING DIAGNOSES: *Caregiver Role Strain; High Risk for Injury; Hypothermia*

ESSENTIAL DISCHARGE CRITERIA

- Is free of symptoms of hypoglycemia
- Maintains consistent oral feeding with demonstrated weight gain
- Maintains normal body temperature
- Parents verbalize and demonstrate knowledge of infant care and list s/s to report to PCP

INFANT OF DIABETIC MOTHER

NURSING DIAGNOSES	OUTCOME CRITERIA	INTERVENTIONS
1 High Risk for Injury (seizures, cerebral damage) *r.t. untreated hypoglycemia*	• Exhibits no s/s of hypoglycemia - irritability, tremors, jittery movements, twitching, seizure activity - cardiac arrest - hypotonia, lethargy - cyanosis, dyspnea, apnea - weak or high pitched cry - hypothermia, diaphoresis - refusal to suck; poor feeding	• Assess on admission for risk factors; if present, implement unit protocol for capillary blood test for glucose • Monitor for s/s of hypoglycemia as indicated • Perform capillary blood glucose testing per unit standard (use warmed heel stick) • Monitor Hct; anticipate reduction transfusion for Hct > 65%
	• Shows serum glucose levels WNL	• Administer ordered glucose therapy; assess effects - provide 5% glucose feeds within 2h of birth if hypoglycemia is suspected or is at risk - expect supportive glucose therapy before s/s appear and in preterm infants - administer ordered glucose infusions; report s/s of hyperglycemic response - monitor for hyperglycemic response in SGA, preterm, low birth weight infants - monitor blood and urine glucose levels to prevent hyperglycemic response - maintain patent infusion line; assess site for extravasation
		RATIONALE: *Adequate circulating glucose is essential to healthy physiologic functioning.*

NURSING DIAGNOSES	OUTCOME CRITERIA	INTERVENTIONS
2 High Risk for Impaired Gas Exchange *r.t. immature pulmonary system, insufficient alveolar surfactant, pulmonary congestion, immature pulmonary system*	• Demonstrates respiratory status within acceptable limits - RR WNL - no expiratory grunting, whining - no nasal flaring - no retractions combined with use of accessory muscles - clear breath sounds - no apnea - no cyanosis in room air - ABGs WNL	• Monitor, manage respiratory status qh, then q2-4h as indicated • Administer warmed O_2 as ordered • Monitor ABGs; report, treat deviations from acceptable levels
		RATIONALE: *The IDM has immature lungs as compared with infant with appropriate gestational age.*
3 Altered Tissue Perfusion (cardiovascular) *r.t. polycythemic hyperviscosity*	• Shows Hct WNL	• Monitor Hct; report deviations; anticipate need for reduction transfusion
	• Shows no hypoglycemia	• Assess blood glucose per unit protocol
	• Displays no plethora	• Assess skin for redness - assess pulses - observe for acrocyanosis
	• Shows no s/s of cardiomegaly - HR, BP, pulses WNL	• Provide continuous cardiopulmonary monitoring • Assess BP and pulses q2-4h as indicated • Assess heart sounds q1-2h
	• Shows no signs of CNS compromise - no lethargy - no hypotonia - no tremulousness - no exaggerated startle - no seizures - no apnea	• Assess infant state, tone, and activity q1-2h as indicated
		RATIONALE: *Polycythemic hyperviscosity impairs circulation to all organs due to sluggish flow.*

NURSING DIAGNOSES	OUTCOME CRITERIA	INTERVENTIONS
4 High Risk for Altered Parenting *r.t. lack of experience with care of ill infant; interruption in bonding process*	• Parents discuss physiology of condition, treatment, rationale; ask appropriate questions	• Teach physiology of condition; encourage questions, discussion
	• Parents list reportable s/s: irritability, twitching, hypotonia, uncoordinated eye or mouth movements	• Describe, provide list of reportable s/s and their significance
	• Parents perform care skills: feeding, diapering, bathing, dressing, soothing infant	• Review and demonstrate normal infant care techniques
	• Parents display bonding behaviors	• Encourage parents to hold, touch, soothe infant
	• Parents possess written follow-up appointments	• Verify possession of follow-up appointments

RATIONALE: *Knowledgeable, competent parents are likely to provide safe, uncomplicated home care.*

OTHER LESS COMMON NURSING DIAGNOSES: *Inability to Sustain Spontaneous Ventilation; Decreased Cardiac Output; Fluid Volume Excess; Altered Nutrition: Less than body requirements; Ineffective Breathing Pattern*

ESSENTIAL DISCHARGE CRITERIA

- Serum glucose and Hct WNL
- Takes, retains 90% of prescribed feedings
- Parents demonstrate skill with infant care and list s/s reportable to PCP

INFECTIOUS DISORDERS

NURSING DIAGNOSES	OUTCOME CRITERIA	INTERVENTIONS
1 High Risk for Infection *r.t. need for indwelling catheters, immaturity, maternal transmission, nosocomial transmission, immune compromise*	• Lab values WNL for age and gestation	• Draw blood work as ordered; discuss results with primary caregiver
	• Cultures are negative	• Administer antibiotics as ordered, according to sensitivities
	• Temperature WNL	• Provide thermal support as indicated • Assess axillary temperature q2h or as indicated • Teach caregivers good hand-washing techniques and strategies to minimize cross-contamination
		RATIONALE: *Assess for infection, minimize potential for transmission.*
2 Ineffective Thermo-regulation *r.t. infectious process, dysmaturity*	• Axillary temperature WNL	• Provide thermal support as indicated - servo control mechanism - double wall isolette - heat shield • Assess environmental and axillary temperature q2h or as indicated
		RATIONALE: *Minimize system compromise due to temperature instability.*
3 Impaired Tissue Integrity *r.t. fluid support, nutrition, biometric monitoring*	• Displays intact skin and mucous membranes	• Use minimal tape • Use monitoring leads appropriate to size and gestation of infant • Remove leads gently
	• IV sites all free of signs of infection	• Assess IV site(s) qh or as indicated • Use aseptic technique when preparing and administering IV fluids and medications • Change IV fluids q24h or per unit standards • Change IV tubing and site per unit standards

NURSING DIAGNOSES	OUTCOME CRITERIA	INTERVENTIONS
		RATIONALE: *Minimize the potential for secondary infection.*
4 Pain *r.t. disease process, medication administration, multiple support measures*	• Demonstrates absence of pain - stable VS, neuro status - responds to comfort measures	• Assess infant status - VS, neuro q2h - stability of HR, respirations, BP • Provide comfort measures, i.e., nesting, pacifier, noise reduction • Administer pain medication as indicated and ordered
		RATIONALE: *Minimize system compromise due to pain stimuli.*
5 High Risk for Infection (transmission) *r.t. contagious nature of virus/bacteria*	• Remains in isolation until free of active virus	• Maintain strict isolation procedures per agency protocol, CDC precautions • Enforce strict hand-washing procedures • Maintain universal precautions
		RATIONALE: *Isolation precautions reduce chance of transmission.*
6 High Risk for Altered Parenting *r.t. infant illness, stress*	• Receives regular visits from parents	• Discuss visiting options with parents/caregivers
	• Receives positive interaction from parents - touching - verbal communication - eye contact	• Teach parents positive interaction strategies relative to infant state, status, and ability to receive stimulation
		RATIONALE: *Provide information, guidance, and support to facilitate taking on parenting role.*

COMP NEONATE

NURSING DIAGNOSES	OUTCOME CRITERIA	INTERVENTIONS
7 Knowledge Deficit *r.t. infant's condition, course and management*	• Parents maintain active involvement in discussion of their infant's care	• Discuss disease process with parents/caregivers • Share expectations for anticipated course • Discuss management strategies as they are implemented or questioned by parents
		RATIONALE: *Minimize parent distress by providing information and inclusion in management process.*

OTHER LESS COMMON NURSING DIAGNOSES: *Parents/Caregivers: Anxiety; Fear; Anticipatory Grieving; Powerlessness; Spiritual Distress; Neonate: Impaired gas exchange; Fluid Volume Deficit; Activity Intolerance; Ineffective Feeding Pattern*

ESSENTIAL DISCHARGE CRITERIA

- Cultures negative; WBC count, platelets, Hb, Hct, clotting factors WNL
- Nutritional intake meets weight gain requirements
- Parents demonstrate skill with infant care and list s/s reportable to primary caregiver

INTRACRANIAL HEMORRHAGE

NURSING DIAGNOSES	OUTCOME CRITERIA	INTERVENTIONS
1 High Risk for Injury (internal) *r.t. prematurity, tissue hypoxia*	• Exhibits no s/s of intracranial hemorrhage - stable, improving LOC - normal fontanel tension - regular respirations - reactive pupils - normal pulse rate	• Assess for s/s of intracranial hemorrhage q8h - sudden deterioration in condition - seizures - decrease in activity - bulging anterior fontanel - irregular respirations, apnea - pupils unreactive to light - bradycardia
	• Shows no increase in head circumference	• Measure head circumference daily
	• Shows normal VS	• Assess VS q2h or as indicated
	• Experiences no events that are associated with abrupt BP changes	• Dilute hypertonic solutions; avoid rapid administration • Organize care to allow sufficient rest/recovery periods • Minimize handling • Prevent hypothermia; conserve body heat • Avoid Trendelenburg's position
		RATIONALE: *Prevent the potential for injury to the neurologic system from increased arterial pressures. Regular monitoring will help establish a baseline to allow for better assessment of changing status.*
2 Impaired Gas Exchange *r.t. prematurity, immature lung tissue, apnea*	• Shows no evidence of hypoxia - blood gases WNL - normal respiratory pattern - no apnea	• Assess respiratory status q2h • Monitor ventilator settings hourly, as indicated • Adapt and minimize procedures and care that may cause hypoxia (two-person suctioning, intubation)
		RATIONALE: *Reduce the likelihood of hypoxia, which causes dilation of cerebral arterioles and thus increases their exposure to arterial pressure.*

NURSING DIAGNOSES	OUTCOME CRITERIA	INTERVENTIONS
3 Knowledge Deficit *r.t. lack of experience with condition*	• Parents verbalize knowledge of physiology of hemorrhage and its treatment	• Explain physiology of intracranial hemorrhage, its causes, course of treatment
	• Parents demonstrate effective care techniques	• Involve parents in infant's care as much as possible; discuss approach/avoidance signals
	• Parents identify sources of support, assistance; and medical follow-up	• Suggest support resources in community • Verify that parents have identified appropriate network for help, family, or community services • Verify that parents have made follow-up appointment with physician
		RATIONALE: *Sharing information will empower parents to be actively involved in decision-making and caregiving.*

OTHER LESS COMMON NURSING DIAGNOSES: *Decreased Cardiac Output; Fluid Volume Deficit; Altered Growth and Development; Ineffective Breathing Pattern*

ESSENTIAL DISCHARGE CRITERIA

- Shows no evidence of increased intracranial pressure
- Shows no apnea of feeding-induced respiratory distress
- Parents demonstrate awareness of referrals/resources
- Parents demonstrate ability to care for infant and list s/s to report to PCP

ISOIMMUNE DISEASE

NURSING DIAGNOSES	OUTCOME CRITERIA	INTERVENTIONS
1 Altered Tissue Perfusion *r.t. decreased C.O.; anemia*	• Shows normal tissue perfusion - no pallor or cyanosis - CRT < 3 sec - stable VS - normal BP - normal skin turgor - normal blood gases	• Note fluid volume overload (excess) • Monitor I&O • Monitor blood gases, CBC, Hct, platelet count, bilirubin, albumin • Weigh daily, same scale • Provide continuous cardiopulmonary monitoring, assess qh and prn - VS - breath sounds - heart tones - CRT • Anticipate need for blood transfusion • Administer IV per order
		RATIONALE: *Tissue perfusion is an indicator of the infant's status. Constant monitoring prompts early detection and management of altered perfusion.*
2 High Risk for Injury (internal) *r.t. thrombocytopenia*	• Shows normal bleeding time; no excessive bleeding	• Monitor heel sticks and venous and arterial punctures for prolonged bleeding • Monitor cord, urine, stools for blood • Monitor infant for s/s of bruising, petechiae, purpura
	• Shows platelets WNL	• Anticipate need for platelet transfusion(s) • Teach parents about potential need for maternal lab work (maternal platelets for infant transfusion) • Monitor lab values q shift
		RATIONALE: *Early detection of bleeding tendencies prompts timely transfusion intervention.*

NURSING DIAGNOSES	OUTCOME CRITERIA	INTERVENTIONS
3 High Risk for Injury (CNS) *r.t. erythroblastosis, hydrops fetalis*	• Shows normal lab values - total and direct bilirubin - Hb, Hct - antigen studies	• Monitor labs: total and direct bilirubin, Hct, spherocytes, antigen • Administer phototherapy as ordered • Anticipate need for exchange transfusion
	• Displays adequate hydration - moist mucous membranes - good skin turgor - normal fontanel tension	• Assess hydration q2h - provide oral care - calculate fluids - monitor I&O
	• Shows CNS function WNL for gestational age	• Assess state, tone, activity, pupils q2-4h • Minimize environmental stimulation - dim lights - decrease noise - nest, position on abdomen • Teach parents "minimal stimulation" strategies
		RATIONALE: *Extravascular hemolysis leads to increased circulating bilirubin which crosses the blood-brain barrier.*

OTHER LESS COMMON NURSING DIAGNOSES: *Decreased Cardiac Output; High Risk for Infection; High Risk for Impaired Skin Integrity; Knowledge Deficit; High Risk for Altered Parenting*

ESSENTIAL DISCHARGE CRITERIA

- Shows normal bleeding time and platelets; has normal Hct, direct and indirect bilirubin
- Gains weight within expected limits
- Exhibits normal infant activity, responsiveness, or parents possess skills for providing care for complex infant
- Parents identify s/s to report to PCP

LARGE FOR GESTATIONAL AGE

NURSING DIAGNOSES	OUTCOME CRITERIA	INTERVENTIONS
1 High Risk for Injury *r.t. hypoglycemia*	• Shows no s/s of hypoglycemia such as - irritability, tremors, jittery movements, twitching, seizure activity - hypotonia, lethargy - cyanosis, dyspnea, apnea - weak or high pitched cry - hypothermia, diaphoresis - refusal to suck	• Assess on admission for risk factors; if present, immediately perform capillary blood test for glucose - use warmed heel stick per unit standard - retest per unit protocol - report deviation from parameters
	• Shows serum glucose levels WNL • Urinary glucose does not exceed trace	• Administer ordered glucose therapy; assess effects - provide formula/breast milk/5% glucose feeds within 2 h of birth if hypoglycemia is suspected or is at risk - expect supportive glucose therapy before s/s appear - administer ordered glucose infusions; report s/s of hyperglycemic response - monitor blood and urine glucose levels to identify glycemic trend - maintain patent infusion line - assess site for extravasation
		RATIONALE: *The LGA infant may be an undiagnosed infant of a diabetic mother.*
2 Impaired Physical Mobility *r.t. fractured clavicle; brachial/facial/phrenic nerve paralysis*	• Displays no residual loss of motion	• Position infant to facilitate correct body alignment • Assess circulation to affected arm, hand • Assess for symmetry of movement; report deviations
	• Displays comfort from pain due to care activities	• Attend to position changes and caregiving activities to minimize pain • Mobilize fractured clavicle per unit standards
		RATIONALE: *LGA infants delivered vaginally are at increased risk for fractured clavicle.*

NURSING DIAGNOSES	OUTCOME CRITERIA	INTERVENTIONS
3 Ineffective Airway Clearance *r.t. neurologic compromise*	• Maintains patent airway	• Assure proper alignment of airway by using prone or side-lying position
	• Handles secretions without respiratory compromise	• Suction prn • Keep bulb/catheter readily available
	• Respiratory effort/rate WNL, no bradycardia	• Provide continuous cardiopulmonary monitoring • Assess RR q1-2h per unit standards
		RATIONALE: *The LGA infant may experience perinatal asphyxia.*
4 Altered Tissue Perfusion *r.t. polycythemic hyperviscosity*	• Manifests Hct WNL	• Monitor Hct, report deviations, anticipate need for reduction transfusion
	• Shows no hypoglycemia	• Assess blood glucose per unit protocol
	• Displays no plethora	• Assess skin for redness • Assess pulses • Observe for acrocyanosis
	• Shows no s/s of cardiomegaly - HR, BP, pulses WNL	• Provide continuous cardiopulmonary monitoring; BP q2-4h as indicated • Assess heart sounds and pulses q1-2h
	• Exhibits signs of CNS compromise - no lethargy - no hypotonia - no tremulousness - no exaggerated startle - no seizures - no apnea	• Assess infant state, tone, and activity q1-2h as indicated • Minimize noxious environmental stimuli
		RATIONALE: *Polycythemic hyperviscosity impairs circulation to all organs due to sluggish flow.*

NURSING DIAGNOSES	OUTCOME CRITERIA	INTERVENTIONS
5 High Risk for Altered Parenting *r.t. lack of experience with ill infant; interruption in bonding process*	• Parents discuss physiology of condition, treatment rationale; ask appropriate questions	• Teach physiology of condition; encourage questions, discussion
	• Parents list reportable s/s: irritability, twitching, hypotonia, uncoordinated eye or mouth movements	• Describe, provide list of reportable s/s and their significance
	• Parents perform care skills: feeding, diapering, bathing, dressing, soothing infant	• Review and demonstrate normal infant care techniques
	• Parents display bonding behaviors	• Encourage parents to hold, touch, soothe infant
	• Parents possess written follow-up appointments	• Verify possession of follow-up appointments

RATIONALE: *Knowledgeable, competent parents are likely to manage home care safely and effectively. Physical closeness and parent-child interaction fosters bonding.*

OTHER LESS COMMON NURSING DIAGNOSES: *Ineffective Feeding Pattern; Decreased Cardiac Output; Interrupted Breastfeeding; Aspiration; Ineffective Thermoregulation; Altered Nutrition: Less than body requirements*

ESSENTIAL DISCHARGE CRITERIA

- Exhibits no s/s of hypoglycemia or plethora
- Takes 90% of prescribed feedings, demonstrates weight gain
- Parents demonstrate skill with infant care and list s/s reportable to PCP

MECONIUM ASPIRATION SYNDROME

NURSING DIAGNOSES	OUTCOME CRITERIA	INTERVENTIONS
1 Impaired Gas Exchange *r.t. pulmonary arteriolar constriction, increased pulmonary vascular resistance, decreased pulmonary blood flow*	• Shows blood gases WNL - PCO_2 levels at lower limits of normal - pH levels at higher limits of normal	• Monitor blood gases as ordered • Adjust inspired O_2 within ordered parameters • Assess continuous pulse oximetry/transcutaneous O_2 monitoring - adjust inspired O_2 within ordered parameters - notify physician of trends
	• Maintains respirations 40-60 bpm - no apnea - no bradycardia	• Assess VS qh or as indicated - provide continuous cardiopulmonary monitoring
		RATIONALE: *Pulmonary arteriolar constriction reduces blood flow to alveoli decreasing gas exchange.*
2 Decreased Cardiac Output *r.t. pulmonary edema, pulmonary arteriolar constriction, fluid shift to interstitial space*	• VS WNL - HR regular - pulse strong	• Provide continuous cardiopulmonary monitoring • Assess VS qh and as indicated • Assess heart sounds q2h
	• CRT < 3 sec -no mottling	• Assess CRT qh • Assess peripheral pulses q4h • Administer IV fluids and vasodilators as ordered
	• Circulating volume WNL	• Monitor I&O - weigh all diapers • Administer volume expanders as ordered - assess CVP, BP qh
		RATIONALE: *Adequate oxygenation facilitates physiologic stability. Asphyxia can damage the cardiac muscle causing altered CO, leading to problems with tissue perfusion, fluid shift to interstitial space, diuresis, and circulatory volume.*

NURSING DIAGNOSES	OUTCOME CRITERIA	INTERVENTIONS
3 Activity Intolerance *r.t. environmental stimulation, CNS irritability*	• Shows no desaturations or bradycardia - quiets with caregiver support	• Provide minimal stimulation environment - respond to alarms promptly - minimize conversation at bedside - hang "quiet" sign - cluster care as tolerated - dim lights or darken room as appropriate - minimize handling of infant - record VS off monitor - use prone or side-lying positioning as indicated • Administer analgesics as indicated
	• Maintains position of comfort	• Nest infant; provide containment - provide sheepskin, gel pillow, wedge
		RATIONALE: *NICU environment is overstimulating especially for very sick infants. Infant physiologic response may place added compromise on the neonate's system.*
4 Altered Renal Tissue Perfusion *r.t. hypovolemia, ischemia, asphyxial renal damage*	• Maintains output WNL	• Maintain strict I&O - weigh diapers • Administer diuretics as ordered
	• Urine chemistries WNL	• Perform urine dip for protein, glucose, leukocytes, Hb
	• Blood chemistries WNL • Peak and trough levels WNL	• Administer nephrotoxic medications (gentamicin) with care - monitor blood levels
		RATIONALE: *During an asphyxial event, blood is shunted away from the kidneys to vital organs increasing the potential for ischemia.*

NURSING DIAGNOSES	OUTCOME CRITERIA	INTERVENTIONS
5 Fluid Volume Excess *r.t. fluid accumulation in pulmonary vessels*	• Shows weight loss of 10% for newborn; weight gain neutral during acute phase	• Monitor and weigh daily, using a bed scale as available
	• Maintains balanced fluids - no edema - serum electrolytes WNL - urinary output WNL	• Administer IV fluids and electrolytes per orders • Assess for edema • Monitor serum electrolytes • Maintain strict I&O - weigh all diapers
	• Produces thin pulmonary secretions, no accumulation - no rales, cyanosis - CVP WNL	• Assess respiratory status qh or as tolerated/indicated - color - breath sounds • Suction as indicated to clear airway • Assess CVP qh or continuously on monitor
		RATIONALE: *Fluid retention is a common complication, primarily in the pulmonary bed.*
6 High Risk for Infection *r.t. debilitation, primary disease*	• Exhibits no signs of sepsis - no apnea, dyspnea - no hypothermia - no pallor, cyanosis - CBC WNL for gestation	• Assess parameters and provide interventions to support infant - continuous cardiopulmonary monitoring - neutral-thermal environment • Monitor blood counts
	• Peak and trough levels WNL	• Administer antibiotics as ordered - monitor peak and trough levels
		RATIONALE: *Neonate is at increased risk for infections. Multiple IV lines increase the risk of nosocomial infection.*

NURSING DIAGNOSES	OUTCOME CRITERIA	INTERVENTIONS
7 **Altered Parenting** *r.t. disease process, interruption of bonding process*	• Parents verbalize understanding of treatment plan	• Provide information - explain disease process - assess coping skills - link with peer support group - provide ongoing updates regarding progress
	• Parents provide care for infant	• Teach parents approach/avoidance signals • Teach parents specialized care
	• Parents verbalize/demonstrate taking in of infant into family	• Promote attachment through role modeling and family trait identification

RATIONALE: *Life-threatening illness places the family at risk for multiple challenges. Communication is essential. Information and role modeling will facilitate taking in by the family.*

OTHER LESS COMMON NURSING DIAGNOSES: *Altered Nutrition: Less than body requirements; Ineffective Thermoregulation; Inability to Sustain Spontaneous Ventilation; Anticipatory Grieving (parents); Altered Urinary Elimination*

ESSENTIAL DISCHARGE CRITERIA

- Takes 90% of feedings and shows consistent weight gain
- Maintains balanced I&O
- Parents demonstrate attachment to infant and skill in performing required care
- Parents have written follow-up instructions/appointments, list s/s to be reported to PCP

NECROTIZING ENTEROCOLITIS

NURSING DIAGNOSES	OUTCOME CRITERIA	INTERVENTIONS
1 High Risk for Infection *r.t. bacterial invasion of necrotic bowel wall*	• Maintains normal, stable axillary temperature	• Assess on admission for high risk factors • Monitor temperature q2h
	• Exhibits no early s/s of NEC such as - gastric aspirates - abdominal distention - apnea/bradycardia - guaiac positive stool	• Measure abdominal girth • Assess for presence of gastric residuals • Initiate NPO for 7-14 day per orders • Assess abdomen: loops of bowel, distention, bowel sounds • Administer antibiotics, IV fluids as ordered • Provide continuous cardio-respiratory monitoring • Perform stool guaiac, Hematest, Clinitest
	• Exhibits no late s/s of NEC such as - lethargy - severe abdominal distention - apnea or bradycardia - pallor or s/s of shock - grossly bloody stools - unstable glucose - unstable Hct	• Insert OG or NG tube; connect to low intermittent suction • Inspect abdomen, measure girth q shift • Assess color, CRT, pulses qh • Provide continuous cardiopulmonary monitoring • Initiate NPO for 7-14 day • Administer antibiotics as ordered • Administer ordered IV therapy • Maintain accurate I&O • Assess blood glucose (heel stick q2-4h) • Monitor Hct • Perform stool Hematest, Clinitest
	• Shows platelets, WBC count, neutrophil count, ABGs WNL	• Monitor lab values and report - increase, decrease in platelet count - increase, decrease in WBC count - decrease in neutrophil count - acidosis

RATIONALE: *Potential for overwhelming sepsis necessitates vigilant observation and thoughtful intervention.*

NURSING DIAGNOSES	OUTCOME CRITERIA	INTERVENTIONS
2 High Risk for Fluid Volume Deficit *r.t. NPO, gastric suction, septic shock*	• Remains adequately hydrated - balanced I&O	• Monitor, maintain hydration - maintain accurate I&O: weigh diapers, measure aspirate, emesis - administer ordered IV fluids - anticipate replacement fluids
	• Maintains normal urinary output - sp. gr. WNL - urine Dipstix WNL	• Monitor urinary output, sp. gr.; Dipstix q2-4h
	• Maintains stable body weight	• Weigh daily, same time, same scale
	• Shows normal serum electrolytes for weight, gestational age	• Monitor serum electrolytes
	• Has moist mucous membranes, good skin turgor, normal fontanel tension	• Inspect mucous membranes, skin, fontanels q2-4h
	• Maintains circulatory volume - CRT < 3 sec	• Monitor CRT q2h • Monitor for increased HR
		RATIONALE: *Adequate circulating volume is essential to maintain good perfusion.*
3 Altered Nutrition: Less than body requirements *r.t. bowel infection*	• Has stable or increasing body weight - 15-30 g/d	• Weigh daily, same time, same scale
	• Tolerates required parenteral nutrition	• Monitor serum electrolytes, blood chemistries • Monitor IV site for patency
	• Exhibits satisfactory GI motility - decreasing gastric residuals - bowel sounds present	• Measure gastric aspirate; replace as ordered • Assess bowel sounds
		RATIONALE: *Adequate nutrition is essential in providing energy for recovery.*

NURSING DIAGNOSES	OUTCOME CRITERIA	INTERVENTIONS
4 High Risk for Injury *r.t. interrupted coagulation processes, sepsis*	• Shows no blood in urine, stools, vomitus	• Assess urine, stools, vomitus for evidence of blood (each specimen)
	• Shows no bleeding, oozing from incisions, infusion sites	• Inspect incisions, infusion sites for oozing as indicated
	• Displays no petechiae, ecchymosis	• Inspect skin for petechiae
	• Shows clotting factors WNL - normal Hb, fibrinogen, platelet levels, CBC, WBC count, differential - normal PT, APTT, thrombin time	• Monitor laboratory values for status of clotting factors; report deviations
	• Has no s/s of septic shock such as - bradycardia or tachycardia - labile BP - extremities hot to touch - CRT > 3 sec	• Monitor, assist to manage s/s of septic shock - maintain patent IV access - monitor VS, BP electronically, continuously - assess extremities for hot, dry skin q2h - assess CRT q2-4h
	• Exhibits no s/s of peritonitis such as - rigid abdomen - bradycardia - hypothermia	• Monitor, assist to manage s/s of peritonitis - assess abdomen hourly or as indicated, including abdominal girth - perform continuous cardiopulmonary monitoring - monitor temperature q2h - limit handling, abdominal palpation - keep patient off abdomen; position side-to-side

RATIONALE: *Complications from NEC can be life-threatening.*

NURSING DIAGNOSES	OUTCOME CRITERIA	INTERVENTIONS
5 **Anxiety** *r.t. life-threatening situational crisis*	• Parents verbalize fears and worries, ask questions, seek information	• Allow time for parents to express feelings - encourage expression of fears, concerns, questions - take extra time to be with parents; be readily available
	• Parents discuss physiology of condition, expected course of treatment, prognosis, s/s that should be reported	• Explain the physiology of NEC, status of infant, expected course, treatment rationale; encourage questions; provide clarification
	• Parents demonstrate required infant care skills	• Demonstrate and explain all routine and special care needs; involve parents in care as appropriate
	• Parents verbalize, express their own and infant's needs without hesitation	• Encourage, assist parents in identifying needs - for comfort, rest, food, support during crisis - finding ways of meeting their own needs - verbalizing perceptions of infant's needs during crisis
		RATIONALE: *NEC can be a life-threatening event of which parents often have no experience in dealing with the concept or the outcomes.*

OTHER LESS COMMON NURSING DIAGNOSES: *Ineffective Thermoregulation; Altered Tissue Perfusion; Impaired Tissue Integrity; Impaired Gas Exchange; Anticipatory Grieving; Activity Intolerance; Ineffective Breathing Pattern*

ESSENTIAL DISCHARGE CRITERIA

- Takes, retains 90% of feedings, consistently gains weight
- Bowel sounds are present, exhibits no abdominal distention
- Parents express confidence in ability to care for infant at home and demonstrate required care techniques
- Parents identify s/s reportable to primary caregiver

PATENT DUCTUS ARTERIOSUS

NURSING DIAGNOSES	OUTCOME CRITERIA	INTERVENTIONS
1 Impaired Gas Exchange *r.t. respiratory distress*	• Exhibits no evidence of respiratory distress - retractions - tachypnea - cyanosis - respiratory acidosis - metabolic acidosis	• Administer O_2 as ordered • Monitor transcutaneous and/or pulse oximetry • Administer assisted ventilation as required • Administer Na bicarbonate as ordered
		RATIONALE: *Pulmonary congestion places the neonate at risk for respiratory distress.*
2 Altered Tissue Perfusion (cardio-pulmonary) *r.t. pulmonary venous congestion, shunting across ductus arteriosus*	• Precordium WNL	• Observe precordial activity q1-2h
	• Has no cardiac murmur • Breath sounds are clear, equal	• Auscultate heart and breath sounds q1-2h
	• Peripheral pulses are nonbounding	• Assess peripheral pulses q2-4h
	• Maintains pulse pressure < 25	• Provide continuous hemodynamic monitoring • Assess BP q1-2h
	• Exhibits closure of ductus arteriosus	• Administer indomethacin as ordered • Monitor urine output • Anticipate need for surgical closure • Discuss treatment plan and its implication with parents
		RATIONALE: *Elevated pulmonary pressures facilitate flow through ductus arteriosus.*
3 High Risk for Fluid Volume Deficit *r.t. diet restriction, fluid restrictions*	• Maintains normal body weight	• Weigh daily, same scale
	• Maintains balanced I&O	• Monitor I&O, sp. gr. q2-4h
	• Shows serum electrolytes WNL	• Monitor serum electrolytes • Administer IV fluids as ordered

NURSING DIAGNOSES	OUTCOME CRITERIA	INTERVENTIONS
	• Shows CRT < 3 sec • Fontanels are flat, soft • Skin turgor WNL	• Assess skin turgor, fontanels, CRT q2-4h
		RATIONALE: *Fluid restriction is used to minimize the effects of pulmonary congestion, yet places the neonate at risk for contracted fluid volume.*

OTHER LESS COMMON NURSING DIAGNOSES: *Altered Growth and Development; Ineffective Infant Feeding Pattern; Ineffective Breathing Pattern*

ESSENTIAL DISCHARGE CRITERIA

- Exhibits no respiratory distress, dyspnea
- Experiences no increased work of breathing with feedings
- Gains $\leq$ 30 g/day
- Takes/retains 90% of feedings
- Parents verbalize home care plans and list s/s reportable to PCP

PERSISTENT PULMONARY HYPERTENSION

NURSING DIAGNOSES	OUTCOME CRITERIA	INTERVENTIONS
1 Decreased Cardiac Output *r.t. pulmonary edema; increased pulmonary vascular resistance*	• Shows normal VS - regular HR - strong pulse	• Assess VS qh • Provide continuous cardiopulmonary monitoring with invasive BP monitoring
	• CRT < 3 sec; no mottling	• Administer IV fluids and vasodilators as ordered • Assess CRT qh • Observe skin color
	• Shows normal circulating volume - balanced I&O - normal urine output - BP WNL	• Monitor I&O • Assess BP at least qh • Administer vasopressors as ordered
		RATIONALE: *Constriction of the pulmonary vasculature decreases available O_2 to the tissues and decreases blood flow to the periphery.*
2 Impaired Gas Exchange *r.t. pulmonary arteriolar constriction, decreased pulmonary blood flow*	• Shows normal blood gases - PCO_2 at lower limits of normal - pH at higher limits of normal - SaO_2 at higher limits of normal	• Monitor blood gases as ordered • Assess continuous pulse oximetry/transcutaneous monitoring • Adjust inspired O_2 within ordered parameters • Notify physician of trends
		RATIONALE: *Respiratory alkalosis may minimize vasoconstriction.*
3 Activity Intolerance *r.t. ventilatory compromise, environmental stimulation*	• Exhibits increasing activity tolerance - no desaturations or bradycardia - quiets with caregiver support	• Provide minimal stimulation environment • Respond to alarms promptly • Minimize conversation at bedside • Hang "quiet" sign • Cluster care as tolerated • Dim lights or darken room as appropriate • Minimize handling of infant • Record VS off monitor

NURSING DIAGNOSES	OUTCOME CRITERIA	INTERVENTIONS
		• Use prone or side-lying positioning as indicated • Administer analgesics as indicated
	• Maintains position of comfort	• Nest infant; provide containment; provide sheepskin, gel pillow, wedge
		RATIONALE: *The NICU environment is overstimulating especially for very sick infants. Infant physiologic responses may place added compromise on the neonate's system.*
4 Fluid Volume Excess *r.t. fluid accumulation in pulmonary vessels*	• Exhibits weight loss of < 10% of birth weight; exhibits neutral weight gain during acute phase	• Monitor and weigh daily, using a bed scale as available
	• Exhibits evidence of balanced fluids - no edema - normal serum electrolytes - normal urine output	• Administer IV fluids and electrolytes per order • Maintain strict I&O; weigh all diapers - check urine for protein, ketones, glucose • Monitor serum electrolytes • Assess for edema
	• Has normal pulmonary secretions; no accumulation of secretions • Has no rales, cyanosis	• Assess, manage respiratory status qh or as indicated - assess color - assess breath sounds - suction as indicated to clear airway
	• Has normal CVP	• Assess CVP qh or continuously on monitor
		RATIONALE: *Fluid retention is a complication of PPHN. The pulmonary bed is a primary site.*

NURSING DIAGNOSES	OUTCOME CRITERIA	INTERVENTIONS
5 High Risk for Infection *r.t. debilitation, primary disease*	• Shows no signs of sepsis - no apnea, dyspnea - no hypothermia - no pallor, cyanosis	• Assess parameters and provide interventions to support infant • Perform continuous cardiopulmonary monitoring • Provide thermoneutral environment
	• Shows normal CBC for gestation	• Monitor blood counts
	• Displays normal peak and trough levels of antibiotics	• Administer antibiotics as ordered; monitor peak and trough levels
		RATIONALE: *The neonate is at increased risk for infection. PPHN may be the result of an infectious process. Multiple IV lines increase the risk of nosocomial infection.*
6 Fear *r.t. disease process; potential death of neonate*	• Parents verbalize understanding of treatment plan	• Provide information • Explain disease process • Assess coping skills • Link with peer support group • Provide ongoing updates re progress
	• Parents provide care for infant	• Teach parents approach/ avoidance signals • Teach parents specialized care
	• Parents verbalize/demonstrate taking in of infant into family	• Promote attachment through role modeling and family trait identification
		RATIONALE: *Life-threatening illness places the family at risk for multiple challenges. Communication is essential. Information and role modeling will facilitate taking in by the family.*

OTHER LESS COMMON NURSING DIAGNOSES: *Ineffective Thermoregulation; Interrupted Breastfeeding; Sleep Pattern Disturbance; Altered Family Processes; High Risk for Altered Parenting; Altered Urinary Elimination; High Risk for Injury; High Risk for Impaired Skin Integrity; Altered Nutrition: Less than body requirements*

ESSENTIAL DISCHARGE CRITERIA

- Is free of compromise to cardiopulmonary system
- Takes 90% of feedings and gains weight consistently
- Maintains balanced I&O
- Parents demonstrate attachment to infant and demonstrate skill in performing required care
- Parents list s/s to be reported to PCP

POSTOPERATIVE CARE

NURSING DIAGNOSES	OUTCOME CRITERIA	INTERVENTIONS
1 Ineffective Breathing Pattern *r.t. perioperative anesthesia*	• Shows stable, normal VS, BP	• Monitor VS, BP q15-30 min until stable, qh as indicated
	• Maintains patent airway	• Maintain airway - keep ETT, resuscitation equipment at bedside - suction prn - keep mechanical ventilation available
	• Is free of s/s of pulmonary compromise - no apneic episodes - no chest retractions - breath sounds clear and equal bilaterally - pink color - pulse oximeter reading WNL - normal blood gases - clear chest x-ray	• Assess for pulmonary compromise q15 min until stable, then qh - administer O_2 as needed per pulse oximeter parameters - x-ray as ordered - turn q2h as tolerated - maintain OG tube to relieve distention and promote adequate air exchange (unless contraindicated) - ABGs as ordered • Assess for central cyanosis, peripheral pallor q15-30 min until stable, then qh - minimize handling - maintain thermoneutral environment
		RATIONALE: *Respiratory compromise is a common problem post-anesthesia, especially in the neonatal population.*
2 High Risk for Fluid Volume Deficit/Excess *r.t. perioperative fluid loss/load*	• Is free of s/s of cardiovascular compromise - regular pulse; 110-160 bpm - urinary output WNL - normal BP - CRT of < 3 sec - no edema	• Assess cardiovascular status q15-30 min until stable, then qh; report deviations from normal limits - monitor apical pulse for irregularities, strength - monitor urinary output - monitor BP - assess CRT qh - assess skin turgor, presence of edema

NURSING DIAGNOSES	OUTCOME CRITERIA	INTERVENTIONS
	• Experiences prompt detection of complications - normal blood gases, Hb, Hct - normal serum Ca, K - normal BUN, creatinine	• Identify complications - monitor blood gases q1-2h or as indicated - monitor Hb, Hct lab results - monitor serum Ca, K for arrhythmia-producing deficits - monitor BUN, creatinine to assess renal function
	• Shows normal circulating volume - balanced I&O - urinary output of at least 0.5-1 mL/kg/h; urinary sp. gr. of 1.003-1.010 - no vomiting; no bright bleeding from operative site	• Monitor, maintain sufficient circulating fluid volume - maintain strict I&O; administer ordered fluid replacements, volume expanders, electrolyte replacements - measure all secretions, excretions, all forms of I&O - monitor urinary output; take sp. gr. q1-2h or as indicated - assess for vomiting and for bright bleeding related to surgical area - assess IV site for redness, edema, infiltration; ensure IV access - monitor BP q1-2h
		RATIONALE: *Fluid shifts may occur during surgery, necessitating close observation during the immediate postoperative period.*
3 Altered Nutrition: Less than body requirements *r.t. hypoglycemia, intolerance to fluid intake, hypocalcemia*	• Shows no weight loss	• Weigh daily • Assess for water retention
	• Is free of s/s of hypoglycemia, hypocalcemia - normal blood glucose and ionized Ca - no prolonged lethargy, flaccidity - no prolonged, intense irritability, tremors - normal gestational status	• Monitor, manage Ca, glucose levels - report deviations - assess activity level for lethargy, hypoglycemia - observe for irritability, tremors associated with hypocalcemia - administer ordered IV glucose, Ca, fluid replacements - provide ordered gavage, TPN
		RATIONALE: *The stress of surgery and the precipitating condition may increase nutritional requirements, yet limit options for adequate calorie/nutrient intake.*

NURSING DIAGNOSES	OUTCOME CRITERIA	INTERVENTIONS
4 High Risk for Altered Parenting *r.t. anxiety, interruption of bonding*	• Parents discuss anatomy of surgery, ask appropriate questions, verbalize realistic perceptions	• Explain, discuss anatomy of the surgery, expected course, treatment rationale; allow for time to listen to fears, concerns
	• Parents visit infant; touch, hold, soothe infant	• Encourage parents to visit as often as possible; allow them to touch, hold, feed as condition permits • Parents demonstrate required infant care techniques
		RATIONALE: *The stress of having a neonate go to surgery may tax the parents' coping beyond their limits of adequate functioning.*
5 High Risk for Infection *r.t. bacterial invasion of surgical site, nosocomial infection*	• Exhibits no redness, edema, purulent drainage at/from incision	• Inspect incisional area for evidence of infection q2-4h prn after initial dressing change by surgeon
	• Displays no s/s of inflammation around insertion site of any chest or other tubes	• Inspect tube, drainage sites for signs of infection: redness, edema, drainage
	• Shows normal, stable axillary temperature	• Monitor axillary temperature electronically or qh until stable, then q2-4h
	• Shows normal WBC count and differential	• Evaluate WBC count, differential for evidence of infection responses
	• Shows negative cultures	• Collect cultures as ordered; evaluate results; report positive cultures • Protect infant from bacterial exposure - maintain strict hand-washing techniques, universal precautions - use sterile techniques for dressing changes, wound care, irrigations
		RATIONALE: *Sick neonates are at high risk for infection due to their poor immunological response.*

NURSING DIAGNOSES	OUTCOME CRITERIA	INTERVENTIONS
6 Pain *r.t. surgical incision, surgery, restriction of movement*	• Is free of s/s of uncontrolled pain - no extended agitation - consolable	• Monitor, manage pain; assess for s/s of pain qh - note agitation, increased HR or BP - provide comfort measures, quiet environment, positioning - administer analgesics per orders; assess effects, side effects
		RATIONALE: *Minimizing pain decreases potential for physiologic compromise due to distress/irritability.*

OTHER LESS COMMON NURSING DIAGNOSES: *Ineffective Airway Clearance; Impaired Gas Exchange; High Risk for Altered Body Temperature; Altered Urinary Elimination; Impaired Skin Integrity; Sleep Pattern Disturbance; Activity Intolerance*

ESSENTIAL DISCHARGE CRITERIA

- Takes, retains 90% of nutrition, with 20-30 g weight gain per day
- Exhibits no respiratory distress on room air
- Parents demonstrate required care techniques and express confidence
- Parents possess follow-up appointments and list s/s reportable to PCP

POST-TERM INFANT

NURSING DIAGNOSES	OUTCOME CRITERIA	INTERVENTIONS
1 Altered Nutrition: Less than body requirements *r.t. increased use of glucose*	• Is free of s/s of hypoglycemia - absence of jitteriness - VS WNL - skin color pink with CRT < 3 sec - infant active; moving extremities - blood glucose WNL	• Perform head-to-toe assessment of infant on admission to nursery and qh for s/s of hypoglycemia • Obtain capillary blood glucose on admission; reassess per unit standard • Assess VS on admission and q2h thereafter
	• Maintains blood glucose WNL	• Obtain serum blood sugar if capillary sample outside of parameters
	• Takes adequate nutrition to maintain blood sugar	• Initiate feeds 2 h after birth or per hospital protocol if infant is without respiratory distress • Initiate IV access per orders for IV glucose administration
		RATIONALE: *Metabolic needs may exceed intake.*
2 Ineffective Thermo-regulation *r.t. decreased liver glycogen, decreased brown fat stores*	• Stabilizes temperature at 36.5-37.5°C (97.8-99.5°F)	• Place newborn in isolette/radiant warmer on admission to nursery as indicated • Assess axillary temperature qh until stable then q2-4h • Delay bath as indicated • Provide warm, humidified O_2, if needed • Dry infant thoroughly • Provide shirt, cap as indicated
	• Maintains cardiopulmonary function WNL	• Assess VS q1-2h until stable • Provide cardiopulmonary monitoring as indicated
	• Exhibits adequate skin perfusion - CRT < 3 sec - skin pink, warm to touch	• Assess CRT and skin perfusion q2-4h
		RATIONALE: *Minimizing heat loss will decrease glucose consumption.*

NURSING DIAGNOSES	OUTCOME CRITERIA	INTERVENTIONS
3 High Risk for Aspiration *r.t. meconium, amniotic fluid aspiration*	• Is free of respiratory distress - VS WNL - color pink with CRT < 3 sec - blood gases WNL - O_2 sat WNL	• At delivery, have emergency equipment functioning at bedside • Perform OPH, NPH bulb suction • Assist with intubation and suctioning below vocal cords • In the nursery: assess lung fields qh until stable • Assess VS and circulation checks q1-2h until stable • Administer warm, humidified O_2 as needed • Monitor pulse oximeter qh • Place on cardiopulmonary monitor as indicated • Monitor blood gases and report to physician
		RATIONALE: *Post-term infants are at increased risk for hypoxia during the birth process, increasing the chance for passage of meconium prior to delivery.*

OTHER LESS COMMON NURSING DIAGNOSES: *Ineffective Airway Clearance; High Risk for Infection; High Risk for Altered Parenting*

ESSENTIAL DISCHARGE CRITERIA

- Blood glucose stabilized WNL, takes 90% of nutrition for growth, gains weight
- Has clear breath sounds with easy respirations, no periodic breathing
- Parents demonstrate required infant care and list s/s to report to PCP

PREOPERATIVE CARE

NURSING DIAGNOSES	OUTCOME CRITERIA	INTERVENTIONS
1 Anxiety *r.t. fear of surgical risks, anesthesia outcomes*	• Parents verbalize acceptance of anesthesia, surgery	• Provide information about anesthesia, surgery - describe type of anesthesia recovery from anesthesia - describe surgery: time to perform, time to recover, visitation of infant post-op
	• Parents verbalize fears, ask questions; make specific plans for time of first post-op visit with infant	• Provide listening, support - encourage to state perceptions - identify, clarify misconceptions - explain that worry is normal - include support persons - verify that parents know of lounges, dining areas, chapel, phones, etc. - let parents know when they can visit before and after surgery
		RATIONALE: *Surgery creates increased anxiety for most persons. These measures will help parents deal with the multiple stressors of having a child undergo surgery.*
2 Knowledge Deficit *r.t. inexperience with surgery, treatment rationale, follow-up care, expected results*	• Parents discuss surgical anatomy; ask questions; express concerns	• Explain surgical anatomy; elicit questions, concerns; clarify misconceptions • Use visual material as available
	• Parents discuss early postoperative course; express appropriate optimism about expected outcomes	• Describe specific medical, nursing activities in first hours post-op: explain rationales for activities
	• Parents hold, cuddle, soothe infant	• Explain how much parents can visit; encourage holding, touching, soothing behaviors as much as possible
	• Parents utilize support persons who are available	• Make referrals to support persons as indicated
		RATIONALE: *This may be the first surgical experience in these parents' lives. Parents may have had information overload, making it difficult to integrate it during the stress of hospitalization.*

3 Fluid Volume Deficit

r.t. NPO; operative condition

NURSING DIAGNOSES	OUTCOME CRITERIA	INTERVENTIONS
	• Is well hydrated - normal BP - HR WNL - balanced I&O - stable body weight - urine output WNL - no vomiting, diarrhea - no evaporative water loss	• Monitor, maintain I&O - assess HR, BP - compare I&O qh - weigh daily, same scale - measure urinary output, weigh diapers, obtain sp. gr. - observe for and record any vomiting, diarrhea - administer ordered parenteral fluids; maintain patent IV - use fluid loss barrier if in radiant warmer
	• Maintains axillary temperature WNL	• Monitor axillary temperature q2-4h or prn - initiate servo control mechanism as indicated
	• Has moist mucous membranes, good skin turgor, normal fontanel tension	• Inspect mucous membranes, skin, anterior fontanel q2h

RATIONALE: *These assessments and interventions minimize potential for occurrence of radiogenic problems associated with dependence on parenteral fluid administration.*

4 High Risk for Infection

r.t. preoperative preparation; preoperative problem

NURSING DIAGNOSES	OUTCOME CRITERIA	INTERVENTIONS
	• Exhibits no evidence of infection - has normal skin color - maintains axillary temperature WNL - is alert and active - exhibits no apnea, bradycardia	• Monitor, manage infection prevention - assess color, noting any pallor or mottling - monitor axillary temperature q2-4h, intervene as indicated - assess activity level, note lethargy - adhere to strict hand-washing - use sterile technique for dressings, irrigations - prohibit contact with persons with URI or other infections

RATIONALE: *Neonates are at increased risk for infection because of their immature immune response.*

NURSING DIAGNOSES	OUTCOME CRITERIA	INTERVENTIONS
5 Altered Nutrition: Less than body requirements *r.t. NPO status, increased nutritional requirements*	• Shows glucose WNL	• Monitor, manage blood glucose - monitor blood glucose levels; report deviations - administer parenteral replacements, TPN per orders, - maintain patent IV as ordered - obtain capillary glucose per unit standard
	• Shows K, Ca, and Na WNL	• Monitor, manage serum Na, Ca, and K - monitor levels; report deviations - administer parenteral replacements, TPN per orders, - maintain patent IV
		RATIONALE: *NPO status limits strategies for meeting nutritional requirements.*

OTHER LESS COMMON NURSING DIAGNOSES: *Inability to Sustain Spontaneous Ventilation; Impaired Tissue Integrity; Impaired Skin Integrity; High Risk for Impaired Skin Integrity; Sleep Pattern Disturbance; Interrupted Breastfeeding; Activity Intolerance*

ESSENTIAL DISCHARGE CRITERIA

- Not applicable

RESPIRATORY DISTRESS SYNDROME

NURSING DIAGNOSES	OUTCOME CRITERIA	INTERVENTIONS
1 Impaired Gas Exchange *r.t. decreased production of surfactant, immature lung tissue* *(Refer to "Assisted Ventilation" care plan)*	• Is free of s/s of respiratory distress - VS WNL - breath sounds clear/equal bilaterally - mild to no retractions - lack of nasal flaring and grunting	• Assess and document q1-2h and prn - temperature, HR, RR, BP - breath sounds - impaired gas exchange: tachypnea, retractions, nasal flaring, grunting, cyanosis, tachycardia, diminished breath sounds, abnormal blood gas values • Maintain patent airway - place small roll under neck - suction airway prn based on secretions and breath sounds
	• Exhibits adequate O_2 perfusion - pink color - blood gases WNL - temperature WNL - HR 110-160 bpm	• Administer O_2 to maintain saturation within parameters • Continuously monitor O_2 saturation per pulse oximetry • Administer exogenous surfactant as ordered • Assess and document blood gas results • Maintain thermoneutral environment • Maintain mean arterial BP WNL • Administer muscle relaxants and sedatives as ordered • Cluster care and minimize handling • Minimize noxious environmental stimuli
		RATIONALE: *Early detection/management of deteriorating respiratory status improve chances that an infant will be able to breathe and maintain optimal blood gas measurements without ventilator assistance.*

NURSING DIAGNOSES	OUTCOME CRITERIA	INTERVENTIONS
2 High Risk for Fluid Volume Excess *r.t. fluid retention first 72 h*	• Shows 10-30 g weight gain per day	• Weigh daily, same scale - use in-bed scales if critical or < 1000 g, as available
	• Maintains balanced I&O, normal electrolytes - serum Na WNL - rapid skin recoil - flat fontanel - moist mucous membranes - VS WNL - urine sp. gr. 1.005-1.020 - 0.5-3 mL/kg/h urine output	• Maintains strict I&O - calculate I&O in mL/kg/h - record intake from all sources - weigh diapers to measure output - indwelling catheter if critical • Monitor urinary sp. gr. q4-8h • Monitor serum electrolytes • Assess and document q2-4h and prn - HR, BP - anterior fontanel status - skin turgor status - mucous membrane status • If infant on radiant warmer bed, cover bed with saran wrap blanket or heat shield • Administer IV fluids per physician orders
		RATIONALE: *Diuresis usually occurs after the first 72 h. Close attention to fluid balance is essential to facilitate recovery.*
3 Altered Nutrition: Less than body requirements *r.t. prematurity and respiratory distress*	• Attains and maintains normal nutritional status as evidenced by weight gain	• Weigh daily, same scale • Maintain caloric intake through intravenous, TPN, or gavage feeding - provide 80-120 kcal/kg every 24 h
	• Maintains normal blood sugar levels	• Monitor for hypoglycemia, especially during stress
	• Maintains balanced I&O - urinary output 0.5-3 mL/kg/h - urinary sp. gr. WNL	• Maintain strict I&O - weigh diapers - monitor sp. gr., Clinitest
	• Maintains normal body temperature	• Keep infant in neutral-thermal environment • Limit unnecessary handling of infant

NURSING DIAGNOSES	OUTCOME CRITERIA	INTERVENTIONS
	• Remains free of signs of GI complications - abdomen without distention, tenderness, discoloration - normal elimination pattern - tolerates enteral feeding	• Monitor for signs of gastrointestinal complications, such as - distress, apnea, bradycardia - constipation/diarrhea - frequent vomiting • Measure residual prior to gavage feedings
		RATIONALE: *Maintenance of sufficient nutrition provides energy and helps to compensate for the high metabolic demands of respiratory distress. Conserving body heat and limiting handling conserve energy and foster weight gain and normal blood glucose levels.*
4 Ineffective Airway Clearance *r.t. presence of ETT or nasal prongs, excessive amount of mucus, atelectasis*	• Displays no respiratory distress - breath sounds clear/equal bilaterally - RR 40-60 bpm - mild to no retractions	• Assess RR and breath sounds q2h and prn - provide continuous cardiopulmonary monitoring • Assess ineffective airway clearance - abnormal breath sounds - tachypnea - retractions - cyanosis - hypoxia • Suction ETT per hospital standards • Reposition q2h and prn
		RATIONALE: *Prevent blocked airway and consequent complications.*

OTHER LESS COMMON NURSING DIAGNOSES: *Altered Nutrition: Less than body requirements; High Risk for Altered Parenting; Dysfunctional Ventilatory Weaning Response; Altered Growth and Development; Knowledge Deficit (parents); High Risk for Infection*

ESSENTIAL DISCHARGE CRITERIA

- Shows no evidence of respiratory distress
- Takes, retains 90% of feedings and consistently gains weight
- Parents verbalize understanding of home care and list s/s reportable to PCP

SEIZURE DISORDER

NURSING DIAGNOSES	OUTCOME CRITERIA	INTERVENTIONS
1 High Risk for Injury *r.t. seizure activity, rapid onset of altered cerebral blood flow*	• Preconvulsive: experiences control of risk factors	• Identify preconvulsive risk factors for seizure disorder - hypoglycemia - perinatal asphyxia - hypocalcemia - infection - congenital abnormalities of CNS - intracranial hemorrhage • Provide continuous cardiopulmonary monitoring • Assess blood sugar per unit protocol • Have suction equipment readily available • Administer O_2 as indicated
	• Convulsive: sustains no external or internal injury during seizure	• Note time, duration, body parts involved and frequency of seizure • Administer medications as ordered - phenobarbital - diazepam - paraldehyde - phenytoin • Maintain patent airway • Ensure patient safety
	• Postconvulsive: experiences safe recovery - VS, BP WNL - clear breath sounds	• Monitor VS per unit standard • Establish a clear airway • Provide oral hygiene
	• Parents discuss, identify safety measures	• Discuss seizure event with parents, treatment, s/s, safety issues

RATIONALE: *Seizures are the most common neurologic problem in the neonatal period and can lead to permanent neurologic damage. Timely intervention can minimize complications.*

NURSING DIAGNOSES	OUTCOME CRITERIA	INTERVENTIONS
2 Ineffective Airway Clearance *r.t. neurologic impairment, immaturity*	• Maintains patent airway	• Suction equipment is readily available and functioning • Position infant to maintain open airway • Teach parents how to use bulb suction
		RATIONALE: *Secretions may block airway during seizure necessitating prompt clearing of airway to facilitate oxygenation.*
3 Ineffective Breathing Pattern *r.t. neuromuscular impairment*	• Lungs clear, breath sounds equal	• Assess breath sounds
	• Respirations easy and WNL	• Assess respiration • Administer O_2 as indicated
	• Demonstrates patent airway	• Position to facilitate patent airway • Provide suction equipment; suction as indicated to clear airway - bulb syringe - catheter
		RATIONALE: *A clear, patent airway facilitates gas exchange and ease of respirations.*
4 Knowledge Deficit *r.t. parents' lack of experience, lack of information about home care*	• Parents demonstrate knowledge of diagnosis and plan of care	• Instruct parents/family regarding the nature of the disorder • Identify previous experience with seizure disorder • Explain diagnostic tests - EEG - Ultrasound - MRI
	• Parents demonstrate understanding of home care management - medication administration - clearing of airway - recognition of seizure activity	• Discuss medications, dose, frequency, purpose, side effects, what to do with missed doses • Encourage family to identify pharmacy for medication refill and to identify "all night" pharmacy in case of emergency

COMP NEONATE

NURSING DIAGNOSES	OUTCOME CRITERIA	INTERVENTIONS
		• Discuss supportive care to be provided during seizure - maintain airway - ensure safety - prohibit anything in mouth - call PCP immediately after event - note activity of muscles, extremities, eyes during event • Discuss plans for home care, babysitters, treatment of seizures that may occur outside of the home
		RATIONALE: *Knowledgeable, competent parents can provide safe, prescribed care.*

OTHER LESS COMMON NURSING DIAGNOSES: *Altered Parenting; Impaired Swallowing; High Risk for Infection; Altered Tissue Perfusion (cerebral, renal)*

ESSENTIAL DISCHARGE CRITERIA

- Maintains patent airway
- Parents demonstrate competence in medication administration and verbalize interventions for seizures
- Takes, retains 90% of feedings
- Parents verbalize plans for follow-up

NURSING DIAGNOSES	OUTCOME CRITERIA	INTERVENTIONS
1 High Risk for Impaired Skin Integrity *r.t. irritation, disruption, breakdown of integument*	• Displays no s/s of skin disorder - localized erythema, warmth - poor turgor, dryness - dry mucous membranes - rashes, irritation, abrasions, breaks - hematoma, petechiae, bruising - abscesses - erythema toxicum	• Monitor high risk infant for s/s of skin disorder q2-4h or as indicated • Decrease potential for skin breakdown - use water-soaked gauze for perineal cleansing - bathe with water only for first week; then 1-2 × week with low alkaline soap - bathe preterm infant with water only and gently pat dry; bathe only when temperature is stable - use sheepskin - use no perfumed products or powder - cleanse oral mucous membranes with water-soaked gauze if NPO - protect from fingernail scratches; apply mittens - use clean, aseptic techniques for skin care • Protect areas of broken skin - expose cord to air and apply antimicrobial ung as ordered - use emollient on cracked skin - determine potential systemic, toxic effects of topical agents before using - cleanse oral mucous membranes with water-soaked gauze if NPO - use porous adhesive skin barrier instead of tape - use Op-site for covering burns, excoriations - rotate or use nonirritating electrodes - rotate IV sites as indicated - inspect for signs of pressure necrosis in infants with immobilized extremity

RATIONALE: *Intact skin and mucous membranes are the first line of defense against infection.*

NURSING DIAGNOSES	OUTCOME CRITERIA	INTERVENTIONS
2 Knowledge Deficit *r.t. special skin care needs*	• Parents discuss importance of good skin care, treatment rationale; ask appropriate questions; perform required skin care	• Provide factual information about skin care; encourage questions; demonstrate required skin care techniques
	• Parents list reportable s/s: fever, abscesses, rash, excoriation, erythema, edema	• Discuss, provide list of reportable s/s
	• Parents possess written follow-up appointments	• Verify possession of follow-up appointments
		RATIONALE: *Parents can provide skin care as a way to bond and to learn how to care for infant.*

OTHER LESS COMMON NURSING DIAGNOSES:
Altered Oral Mucous Membrane; High Risk for Infection

ESSENTIAL DISCHARGE CRITERIA

- Parents demonstrate required skin care techniques
- Parents list reportable s/s to PCP

SMALL FOR GESTATIONAL AGE

NURSING DIAGNOSES	OUTCOME CRITERIA	INTERVENTIONS
1 Ineffective Thermo-regulation *r.t. reduced body fat, prematurity, absent brown fat*	• Shows VS stable WNL for GA/wgt - no nasal flaring, retractions - no hypotension	• Provide continuous cardiopulmonary monitoring • Monitor VS, BP q30-60 min until stable, then q1-2h per unit standard
	• Shows no s/s of hypothermia - no mottling, pallor, coolness of skin	• Prevent, alleviate hypothermia by providing thermoneutral environment - keep nursery temperature stable at 77°F (25°C) - prevent drafts, cold equipment, wet linens - provide plastic wrap, blanket, or heat shield - provide humidity - alleviate hypothermia by using incubator, radiant warmer - initiate servo control mechanism
		RATIONALE: *Reduced body fat decreases available glucose stores and reduces insulation from heat loss.*
2 High Risk for Fluid Volume Deficit *r.t. sensible and insensible fluid loss*	• Maintains stable body weight	• Weigh daily, same scale • Monitor and administer ordered fluids, electrolytes; assess effects
	• Shows urinary sp. gr. WNL	• Assess urinary sp. gr. q2-4h
	• Shows no glycosuria	• Assess for glucosuria q4-8h
	• Shows Na, K levels WNL	• Monitor electrolyte panels for Na, K changes; report deviations
		RATIONALE: *The SGA infant has decreased reserves and is sensitive to small deviations from normal.*

NURSING DIAGNOSES	OUTCOME CRITERIA	INTERVENTIONS
3 Altered Nutrition: Less than body requirements *r.t. inadequate stores of glycogen, Ca, iron*	• Maintains body weight (increases or remains stable)	• Weigh daily, same scale • Progress feedings as tolerated per orders
	• Shows no s/s of hypoglycemia - no lethargy, flaccidity - blood glucose WNL for GA	• Monitor for hypoglycemia - assess lethargy, poor muscle tone, flaccidity q2-3h - monitor blood glucose levels
	• Shows no s/s of hypocalcemia - no hyperactivity, irritability, tremors - serum Ca WNL for GA	• Monitor for hypocalcemia - observe for irritability, tremors - monitor serum Ca levels
	• Takes, retains required calories, nutrition - no vomiting, diarrhea	• Calculate caloric requirements - monitor rate of compliance q2-3h; report deviations - administer ordered IV glucose, Ca, TPN - perform ordered gavage - progress to breast/bottle feedings as indicated
		RATIONALE: *The SGA infant has an increased metabolic rate and therefore increased caloric need while at risk potential for fluid overload.*
4 High Risk for Infection *r.t. immature immune system, intrauterine exposure*	• Is free of infection - body temperature WNL for GA/wgt - CBC WNL - no conjunctivitis, skin rashes, localized lesions, purpura	• Monitor, prevent infection - initiate universal precautions - assess body temperature q2h - monitor blood counts for evidence of infection - inspect eyes, skin for inflammation (rashes, lesions) - maintain strict hand-washing, gowning, masking, gloving - restrict staff, visitors with infections
		RATIONALE: *The infant may be SGA due to a viral infection.*

NURSING DIAGNOSES	OUTCOME CRITERIA	INTERVENTIONS
5 Impaired Gas Exchange (high risk for) *r.t. polycythemia, respiratory infection*	• Maintains respiratory status within acceptable limits - RR WNL - no expiratory grunting, - no nasal flaring, retractions with use of accessory muscles - no apnea - no cyanosis in room air - clear breath sounds - ABGs WNL	• Monitor, manage respiratory status qh × 8h, then q2-4h as indicated - use pulse oximeter and/or transcutaneous monitor; initiate immediate treatment if deviations occur - monitor serial ABGs; report, treat deviations from acceptable levels - detect, manage apneic episodes; place apneic infants on apnea monitor
		RATIONALE: *The SGA infant will have respiratory compromise due to infectious process or poor pulmonary blood flow.*
6 Sensory/ Perceptual Alterations (all senses) *r.t. intensive care environment*	• Displays no evidence of hypo- or hyperactive responses - looks at, responds to large objects - no sighing, turning away - turns head toward sounds - no absence of response, apnea, or bradycardia - displays no inappropriate crying or responding only to painful or excess stimuli - displays hand-to-mouth activities - displays no hyperactivity or hypoactivity	• Monitor, manage level of hypo- or hyperactive responses in an individualized manner - provide containment, nesting - provide visual stimulation with large black and white object 8 inches from eyes, per infant cues - hold upright providing eye contact - avoid bright, harsh lights - reduce excessive, repetitive, ambient sounds if possible - provide auditory stimulation (talk to infant, call by name, play tapes, music) - provide tactile stimulation as condition permits (stroking of entire body; hold, cuddle, caress cheeks; touch with various textured fabrics) - feed, provide pacifier for sucking and gustatory stimulation - change position q2h; avoid supine position
	• Sleeps, naps at appropriate intervals for condition, GA	• Plan care to provide uninterrupted periods for rest, sleep
	• Parents are actively involved in behavioral-based care	• Teach parents approach and avoidance cues, reinforce behavioral-based care strategies
		RATIONALE: *The SGA infant is often irritable, therefore close attention to minimizing environmental stress is necessary.*

NURSING DIAGNOSES	OUTCOME CRITERIA	INTERVENTIONS
7 Anxiety *r.t. lack of experience with care of immature infant at home*	• Parents verbalize concerns; discuss physiology of prematurity, treatment rationale; ask questions	• Assess, provide information - assess parents' level of anxiety and use of coping mechanisms - provide factual information about prematurity; encourage questions - provide ongoing information about infant's progress - refer to support group
	• Parents perform holding, feeding, dressing, diapering, soothing, developmental strategies	• Demonstrate holding, feeding, soothing, dressing, diapering techniques; involve parents in caregiving as condition permits
	• Parents perform required care procedures	• Describe, demonstrate required care techniques
	• Parents list reportable s/s: weight loss or no gain, poor feeding, fever, dyspnea, lethargy, twitching, tremors	• Describe, provide list of reportable s/s
	• Parents express confidence in ability to manage at home; possess written follow-up appointments for well-child care	• Facilitate planning for home care - refer to community resources as needed - explain need for well-child care - verify possession of follow-up appointments
		RATIONALE: *Knowledgeable, competent parents are likely to provide for safe, uncomplicated home care.*

OTHER LESS COMMON NURSING DIAGNOSES: *Altered Tissue Perfusion; Activity Intolerance; Ineffective Breathing Pattern; Fatigue; Hypothermia*

ESSENTIAL DISCHARGE CRITERIA

- Takes 90% of prescribed feedings, fluids
- Achieves consistent weight gain
- Parents perform required care techniques
- Parents list reportable s/s and possess written follow-up appointments

SPINA BIFIDA

NURSING DIAGNOSES	OUTCOME CRITERIA	INTERVENTIONS
1 Impaired Skin Integrity *r.t. presence of sac, paralysis, continual dribbling of urine and feces* *(Refer to "Preoperative" care plan)*	• Shows no signs of skin breakdown or excoriation	• Protect meningeal sac from injury until surgical repair • Maintain hip and lower extremity in anatomically correct position, provide ROM q4-8h • Discuss with parent methods of protecting infant from skin breakdown • Turn child q2h, side, prone, side • Use sheepskin and nesting • Do head-to-toe skin checks q4-8h
	• Perianal area remains clean and dry	• Observe, report, and record characteristics of anal opening and stool pattern • Clean perineum as soon as possible after each soiling, pat dry • Apply appropriate ointment or cream around the perineal region • Leave excoriated areas open to air as much as possible
		RATIONALE: *Decreased sensation and movement in extremities and poor circulation make the infant vulnerable to skin breakdown. Positioning, skin care, and protective measures are necessary to prevent pressure or injury.*
2 High Risk for Infection *r.t. open sac with draining, protruding spinal contents* *(Refer to "Postoperative" care plan)*	• Shows VS WNL	• Assess VS q2-3h; report deviations from normal
	• Shows WBC count WNL; cultures negative	• Monitor laboratory results
	• Meningeal sac/repair incision remains clean, intact, and exhibits no signs of infections	• Observe, report, and record any s/s of infection, including foul-smelling urine, elevated temperature, and cloudy urine • Position infant to prevent sac/incision contamination from urine and stool • Apply sterile moist dressings as ordered

COMP NEONATE

NURSING DIAGNOSES	OUTCOME CRITERIA	INTERVENTIONS
		• Administer antibiotics as ordered • Avoid urethral contamination with stool • Facilitate good hand-washing for staff and family **RATIONALE:** *Close observation for signs of infection allows early detection and treatment to reduce the potential for complications.*
3 Altered Tissue Perfusion (cerebral) *r.t. hydrocephalus, increased intracranial pressure* *(Refer to "Hydrocephalus" care plan)*	• Exhibits no signs of increased intracranial pressure	• Assess and report signs of increased intracranial pressure: fontanel tension, LOC, lethargy, change in VS, seizures, pupillary changes, vomiting • Assess neurologic status q2-4h • Measure head circumference daily or as ordered **RATIONALE:** *Changes in neurologic status are indicative of altered perfusion.*
4 Impaired Physical Mobility *r.t. lower extremity paralysis, postoperative immobility*	• Maintains physical mobility	• Perform ROM to extremities daily • Use proper positioning with pillow, rolls, wedge, splints • Refer to physical therapy for assessment, intervention **RATIONALE:** *Passive and active ROM of muscles increase circulation and maintain joint mobility. Active motion helps maintain muscle strength and prevent atrophy of muscles.*

NURSING DIAGNOSES	OUTCOME CRITERIA	INTERVENTIONS
5 Urinary Retention *r.t. lack of nerve innervation, urination*	• Has no urinary retention	• Assess bladder, perform Credé's method per protocol • Intermittent clean catheterization as ordered
		RATIONALE: *Frequent monitoring of urination prompts early detection and management.*
6 Bowel Incontinence *r.t. lack of nerve innervation for defecation*	• Has no diarrhea or constipation	• Monitor stools for color and consistency • Administer antidiarrheal medications as ordered
		RATIONALE: *Frequent monitoring of bowel continence prompts early detection and management.*
7 Altered Growth and Development *r.t. hospitalization, extent of defect*	• Demonstrates consistent weight gain	• Weigh daily, same scale
	• Takes adequate nutritional intake to meet caloric needs for normal growth and development	• Maintain IV solutions as ordered • Advance to breast milk/formula as ordered • When fed in prone position, turn to side, elevate head • Assess sucking capabilities
	• Demonstrates behaviors consistent with gestational age and chronological age	• Provide child with auditory, tactile, vestibular, and sensory stimulation • Assist parents to make informed decisions about plan of care • Make referrals to appropriate developmental program • Instruct parents on normal infant development
		RATIONALE: *Stimulation enhances the child's physical, emotional, and mental development. Children with meningomyelocele and hydrocephalus are at risk for neurologic problems and developmental delays.*

NURSING DIAGNOSES	OUTCOME CRITERIA	INTERVENTIONS
8 High Risk for Altered Parenting *r.t. separation from the infant, hospitalization at birth*	• Parents/family visit regularly; hold, interact, provide care for infant • Engages in caretaking activities, exhibiting attachment behaviors	• Encourage parents/family to participate in care activities and to express feelings and concerns
	• Family understands the complexities of ongoing care • Family members adjust to idea of child needing extensive long-term care	• Explain to parents the nature of the defect and what they may expect during hospitalization
	• Families able to verbalize feelings and use resources appropriately	• Encourage family to contact local/national Spina Bifida Association
		RATIONALE: *Early family involvement enhances acceptance of extent of care needed.*
9 Knowledge Deficit *r.t. lack of information about condition, treatment, and home care*	• Parents verbalize understanding of child's condition, treatment, follow-up appointments, and home care instructions	• Plan teaching according to parent's needs • Assess family's level of understanding of health concerns and any new routines: ROM, diet, or splints • Familiarize family with community resources • Initiate home visits as appropriate • Allow practice of needed skills • Emphasize the importance of follow-up appointment and care
		RATIONALE: *Assessment of learning needs and developmental level is essential in providing appropriate information. Knowledge of care needed at home increases compliance with treatment plan.*

OTHER LESS COMMON NURSING DIAGNOSES: *Hypothermia; Potential for Injury; Altered Family Process; Altered Nutrition: Less than body requirements; Ineffective Airway Clearance; Inability to Sustain Spontaneous Ventilations*

ESSENTIAL DISCHARGE CRITERIA

- Skin is dry, intact; incision healing
- Takes 90% of nutritional requirements
- Family is familiar with community resources
- Family is able to perform routine daily care
- Family is able to recognize changes in child's neurologic status
- Family is able to monitor I&O
- Parents possess follow-up appointments

TALIPES (CLUB FOOT)

NURSING DIAGNOSES	OUTCOME CRITERIA	INTERVENTIONS
1 High Risk for Injury (foot deformity) *r.t. delayed identification, treatment of talipes deformity*	• Experiences early detection of talipes deformity	• Examine flexion, turning, and general position of foot and toes • Test mobility, flexibility of foot and toes
	• Parents discuss anatomy of deformity, rationale for cast, splint	• Anticipate casting or splint; explain rationale to parents
		RATIONALE: *Early identification of deformity allows prompt intervention to minimize loss of function.*
2 High Risk for Injury (neurovascular damage) *r.t. irritation, redness, abrasions associated with irritation from cast, splint edges; prolonged pressure from cast, splint; pressure, constriction from tight cast, splint*	• Displays no coolness, pallor, pulselessness, loss of sensation in lower extremity	• Inspect, test lower extremity for neurovascular changes q2h - palpate pedal pulses - perform CRT test of nail beds - do pinprick test - feel for coolness of leg, foot, toes - inspect for pallor of leg, foot, toes
	• Shows no evidence of tightness, skin abrasions around cast edges; no redness, excoriation, abrasions	• Protect skin - if casted, use foam padding around legs - turn infant q2h; use pillows for supports
		RATIONALE: *Minimize potential for skin breakdown and/or neurovascular compromise.*
3 Knowledge Deficit *r.t. splinting, casting of foot*	• Parents discuss anatomy of deformity; acknowledge that they will provide consistent follow-up	• Explain anatomy of deformity - draw diagrams of anatomy of dislocation - remind that treatment is lengthy, consistency is key to success
	• Parents list reportable s/s: absent pedal pulses; pallor, coolness of toes, nail beds; loss of sensation, feet, toes	• Describe potential complications of casting, splinting; describe, provide list of reportable s/s
	• Parents perform proper care techniques; splinting, cast care	• Demonstrate required special care

NURSING DIAGNOSES	OUTCOME CRITERIA	INTERVENTIONS
	• Parents possess written follow-up appointments	• Verify follow-up appointments for cast, splint care, skin care **RATIONALE:** *Knowledgeable, competent parents are likely to provide the effective long-term care that is required.*

OTHER LESS COMMON NURSING DIAGNOSES: *High Risk for Impaired Skin Integrity; Altered Tissue Perfusion; Altered Growth and Development; High Risk for Altered Parenting*

ESSENTIAL DISCHARGE CRITERIA

- Displays clear, intact skin
- Displays no pallor, coolness of feet, toes, nail beds
- Has intact pedal pulses
- CRT of toes, nail beds is < 3 sec
- Parents demonstrate correct care techniques
- Parents possess written follow-up appointments

THERMAL INSTABILITY

NURSING DIAGNOSES	OUTCOME CRITERIA	INTERVENTIONS
1 Ineffective Thermo-regulation *r.t. prematurity, infection, ambient temperatures, hypothermia, hyperthermia*	• Maintains body temperature WNL	• Monitor body temperature - monitor axillary temperatures q30-60 min x 2h, then 2-4h - use servo control mechanism as indicated
	• Exhibits HR, respirations, BP, WNL • Displays no nasal flaring, retractions	• Monitor HR, respirations, BP q30-60 min until stable and WNL, then q2-4h per unit standard
	• Displays no mottling, pallor, coolness	• Assess skin color and temperature • Alleviate hypothermia; use radiant warmer, incubator, thermal shield, provide servo control mechanism
	• Displays no tremors, irritability, twitching, seizures; no warmth, flushing, diaphoresis of skin	• Alleviate hyperthermia; decrease ambient temperature, unbundle, provide servo control mechanism
	• Experiences required ambient nursery temperature; no drafts, cold equipment, wet linens	• Maintain thermoneutral environment - keep nursery temperature stable at 77°F (25°C) - prevent drafts - use warm equipment - keep linens dry
		RATIONALE: *Thermal compromise places the infant at risk for physiologic distress, i.e., hypoglycemia, respiratory distress.*
2 High Risk for Injury (hypoxia) *r.t. cold stress; hypoxia, hypoglycemia, acidosis*	• Shows no s/s of cold stress - temperature WNL - no mottling, pallor - no central cyanosis, cold skin - no irritability and restlessness followed by lethargy, flaccidity, feeble reflexes, feeble cry - no slow, shallow irregular respirations with expiratory grunt - no bradycardia	• Warm slowly: no > 1°C per hour - swaddle, dress, cap as indicated - keep ambient temperature warmer than skin per unit guidelines - administer ordered warmed, humidified O_2 - administer ordered volume expander, Na bicarbonate • Provide continuous pulse oximetry, cardiopulmonary monitoring
	• Shows no s/s of hypoglycemia; serum electrolytes WNL	• Monitor serum glucose, serum electrolytes; report deviations
		RATIONALE: *Cold stress increases metabolic rate and O_2 consumption.*

NURSING DIAGNOSES	OUTCOME CRITERIA	INTERVENTIONS
3 Knowledge Deficit *r.t. lack of experience with thermoregulation needs*	• Parents discuss physiology of condition, temperature control, special warming procedures; expected course of treatment; ask appropriate questions	• Explain physiology of thermoregulation; encourage questions, discussion
	• Parents demonstrate required thermal protective measures when holding, feeding, visiting infant	• Explain, demonstrate care techniques: protective clothing, covering, cap, external heat source, avoid drafts
	• Parents perform axillary temperature-taking; make accurate readings	• Demonstrate how to take and read axillary temperature

RATIONALE: *Parents attention to temperature needs can minimize infants risk for infection, respiratory distress, feeding problems.*

OTHER LESS COMMON NURSING DIAGNOSES: *High Risk for Altered Parenting; Ineffective Infant Feeding Pattern; Impaired Gas Exchange; Hypothermia; Hyperthermia; High Risk for Infection*

ESSENTIAL DISCHARGE CRITERIA

- Maintains core and skin temperatures
- Serum glucose, Na, K WNL
- Has lusty cry and pink, moist mucous membranes
- Takes, retains at least 90% of prescribed feedings, fluids
- Parents demonstrate required thermal protective techniques
- Parents demonstrate ability to take, read, and evaluate axillary temperature
- Parents possess written follow-up appointments

TRACHEOESOPHAGEAL FISTULA

NURSING DIAGNOSES	OUTCOME CRITERIA	INTERVENTIONS
1 Ineffective Airway Clearance *r.t. regurgitation through esophagus/ trachea to trachea, mouth, and nose*	• Maintains patent airway - minimal amounts of collecting secretions - no episodes of aspiration	• Monitor, manage airway clearance - maintain NPO - keep suction, O_2, ETT, resuscitation equipment available - suction OPH prn - insert replogle into blind pouch, connect to suction per orders - position on side with HOB elevated - record amount and character of secretions
	• Exhibits normal respiratory status - no choking, coughing, regurgitation through mouth and nose - RR WNL - no grunting, retractions, use of accessory muscles - no nasal flaring; no cyanosis - clear breath sounds - pink color - blood gases within normal parameters - O_2 sats WNL - clear chest x-ray	• Monitor, manage supportive respiratory therapy - attach ordered gastric decompression tube to straight suction - assess rate, depth, effort; retractions; nasal flaring - observe color, HR, activity - monitor blood gases - monitor serial x-rays - administer mechanical ventilation and O_2 therapy per orders - monitor pulse oximeter as ordered
		RATIONALE: *High risk for respiratory compromise due to communication TEF.*
2 High Risk for Fluid Volume Deficit *r.t. NPO; gastric suction*	• Remains adequately hydrated - balanced I&O - urinary output 0.5-3 mL/kg/h - urine sp. gr. 1.005-1.015 - HR & BP WNL	• Monitor, maintain hydration - assess VS q1-2h - maintain strict I&O - weigh diapers; measure aspirate, emesis - monitor urinary sp. gr. q2-4h - administer ordered IV fluids, nutrition - maintain patent IV as ordered
	• Maintains axillary temp 36.4°–37.6°C (97.5°-99.7°F)	• Minimize evaporative heat loss by use of isolette, heat shield
	• Shows serum electrolytes WNL for weight, gestational age	• Monitor serum electrolytes
	• Has moist mucous membranes, good skin turgor, normal fontanel tension	• Inspect mucous membranes, skin, fontanels q2-4h

NURSING DIAGNOSES	OUTCOME CRITERIA	INTERVENTIONS
		RATIONALE: *TEF requires surgical repair; therefore, attention to fluid volume reduces operative risks.*
3 Altered Nutrition: Less than body requirements *r.t. NPO; gastric suction; feeding intolerance*	• Shows stable or < 10% weight loss	• Weigh daily, same scale
	• Takes required parenteral, gastrostomy nutrition - has gastric residual < 10% of feeding - no increase in abdominal girth, no distension - no regurgitation	• Provide required nutrition - administer TPN per orders - graduate from small, dilute feedings to greater volume, strength as tolerated - aspirate, measure gastric residual - provide pacifier to meet sucking needs
		RATIONALE: *The use of oral or gastrostomy feedings are dependent on response to surgery and initial feedings.*
4 Knowledge Deficit *r.t. lack of experience with care of infant; information regarding correction of deficit*	• Parents verbalize feelings, concerns	• Encourage expressions of feelings, fears
	• Parents discuss physiology of condition, ask appropriate questions	• Provide information about infant's status and expected recovery period
	• Parents display bonding behaviors; participate in care as appropriate to condition	• Foster parent-infant contact - encourage parents to visit, touch, hold, feed infant depending upon condition - explain, demonstrate required care techniques
	• Parents identify needed resources	• Provide home care resources - refer parents to community resources for home care supervision - refer to social services as needed
	• Parents possess written follow-up appointments	• Verify possession of follow-up appointments
		RATIONALE: *Maximize parent information, involvement, and care to encourage acceptance and provision of necessary care at home.*

OTHER LESS COMMON NURSING DIAGNOSES: *Ineffective Breathing Pattern; Impaired Gas Exchange; High Risk for Aspiration; High Risk for Infection; High Risk for Altered Parenting*

ESSENTIAL DISCHARGE CRITERIA

- Tolerates/retains 90% of feedings and gains weight
- Incision healing, without drainage
- Shows no respiratory compromise
- Parents demonstrate required care techniques and lists s/s reportable to PCP

TRANSIENT TACHYPNEA OF THE NEWBORN

NURSING DIAGNOSES	OUTCOME CRITERIA	INTERVENTIONS
1 Ineffective Airway Clearance *r.t. diminished alveolar surfactant; alveolar airway obstruction; retained lung fluid; alveolar collapse; atelectasis*	• Maintains respiratory status within acceptable limits - normal RR - no apnea - no expiratory grunting, wheeze - no nasal flaring, retractions, use of accessory muscles - clear breath sounds - no pallor, cyanosis - normal HR, BP	• Assess respiratory status qh until stable, then q2-4h as indicated • Monitor VS qh, then q1-4h as indicated • Provide continuous cardiopulmonary monitoring • Assess for changes in activity levels • Suction as needed to maintain clear airway • Inspect for cyanosis qh or as ordered
	• Shows normal serial ABGs	• Monitor serial ABGs; report deviations • Administer warmed, humidified O_2 as ordered
	• Airway is patent	• Inspect x-ray for air bronchograms • Suction as indicated
		RATIONALE: *TTN is often transitory, associated with cesarean delivery and transient pulmonary edema.*
2 High Risk for Fluid Volume Deficit *r.t. NPO, gastric suction*	• Maintains balanced I&O - no decrease in body weight (< 10% of BW) - urinary output WNL	• Monitor, manage I&O - weigh qd, same scale - monitor urinary sp. gr. q2-4h
	• Maintains normal body temperature for gestational age, weight	• Monitor body temperature q2-4h
	• Shows normal serum electrolytes for weight, gestational age	• Monitor serum electrolytes • Administer IV fluids as ordered
	• Displays moist mucous membranes, good skin turgor	• Inspect skin, mucous membranes
	• Has normal fontanel tension	• Inspect fontanels q4h
		RATIONALE: *Infants with TTN are NPO until RR is 60-80 bpm, depending on institutional standards.*

NURSING DIAGNOSES	OUTCOME CRITERIA	INTERVENTIONS
3 High Risk for Altered Parenting *r.t. separation, interruption in bonding process; lack of experience with care of infant with pulmonary complications*	• Parents verbalize feelings, concerns	• Encourage expressions of feelings, fears
	• Parents discuss physiology of condition, ask appropriate questions	• Provide information about infant's status and expected recovery period
	• Parents display bonding behaviors; participate in care as appropriate to condition	• Foster parent-infant contact - encourage parents to visit, touch, hold, feed infant depending upon condition - explain, demonstrate required care techniques
	• Parents possess written follow-up appointments	• Verify possession of follow-up appointments

RATIONALE: *Interruption in the normal infant integration process produces anxiety and need for information.*

OTHER LESS COMMON NURSING DIAGNOSES: *Interrupted Breastfeeding; Fatigue; Altered Nutrition: Less than body requirements; Ineffective Thermoregulation; Ineffective Breathing Pattern; Impaired Gas Exchange*

ESSENTIAL DISCHARGE CRITERIA

- Has normal RR, depth, character; has normal PCO_2 and PO_2
- Takes, retains 90% of required nutrition and demonstrates weight gain
- Parents demonstrate required care techniques
- Parents possess written follow-up appointments

VERY LOW BIRTH WEIGHT INFANT

NURSING DIAGNOSES	OUTCOME CRITERIA	INTERVENTIONS
1 Ineffective Thermo-regulation *r.t. thin skin, minimal subcutaneous fat, immature thermoregulatory system*	• Maintains normal axillary temperature (36.5-37.2°C)	• Assess axillary temperature q1-4h and prn • Maintain thermoneutral environment - radiant warmer - double-walled incubator or single-walled incubator with inner heat shield - use servo control mechanism with probe attached to infant's epigastric area if possible (not over bone) • Record isolette temp with each recording of temperature • Cover open bed of radiant warmer with plastic wrap or provide heat shield • Use external heat source during procedures, placed about 28 in from infant • Bathe only when necessary • Place cap/booties on infant unless contraindicated • Provide warmed humidity (50-80%) to covered radiant warmer bed or incubator • Organize nursing care to avoid unnecessary fluctuation in environmental temperature
	• Maintains stable O_2 requirements	• Monitor pulse oximetry O_2 hourly prn • Assess respiratory status qh
		RATIONALE: *Providing a thermoneutral environment minimizes O_2 consumption and prevents complications of hypothermia and hyperthermia.*
2 Activity Intolerance *r.t. prematurity, immature CNS*	• Maintains stable O_2 requirements	• Provide pulse oximetry monitoring • Modify environment - decrease light and noise at bedside/room - cover isolette with blanket - use radiant warmer covers

NURSING DIAGNOSES	OUTCOME CRITERIA	INTERVENTIONS
	• Tolerates activity with minimal fluctuation in HR, RR, BP, muscle tone	• Cluster nursing care; provide rest periods during care as needed • Provide continuous cardiopulmonary monitoring
	• Shows decrease in appearance of stress signals in response to activity	• Assess infant for "stress cues" during activity (stop activity if present) - tachypnea/apnea - tachycardia - worsening of color - gagging, emesis - twitches, startles - frantic activity - flaccid posture - hyperextension of extremities - arching - rapid transitions between states or decreased range of states • Provide minimal handling; evaluate importance of any activity before proceeding • Position prone or side-lying; nest with blanket rolls around sides, back, feet, and head to contain extremities • Document tolerance to activity and successful interventions
		RATIONALE: *These measures protect infant from overstimulation.*
3 High Risk for Impaired Skin Integrity *r.t. mechanical factors, immature skin, immobility*	• Has no pressure ulcers, burns, bruises, or excoriations	• Assess skin and mucous membranes every 2 to 4h and prn; notify physician of changes • Reposition every 2 to 4h unless contraindicated; assess pressure areas • Slowly and gently perform passive ROM at least every 4h as needed and as tolerated • Handle infant's skin with extreme care; educate auxillary caregivers (lab, radiology) to do so also

NURSING DIAGNOSES	OUTCOME CRITERIA	INTERVENTIONS
		• Minimize use of tape; use pectin-based barrier between tape and skin • Avoid use of skin preparations or adhesive removers; use water to loosen tape • Bathe only when needed using warm water; use sterile water if skin broken down • Provide routine oral care with sterile H_2O for NPO patients • Rinse off topical disinfectants immediately after procedures to prevent chemical burns and absorption • Assess IV sites at least qh and discontinue IV at first sign of infiltration • Avoid use of hot water bottles or gloves and chemical heating devices directly on the skin • Use pulse oximetry instead of transcutaneous O_2 monitors when possible; if TCM used, site should be changed frequently (q1-2h) and reliable lowest heat setting used • Provide 50-80% humidity to covered bed of radiant warmer or isolette • Avoid use of lotions, creams, powder • Position infant on covered sheepskin/lambswool or water mattress
		RATIONALE: *Intact skin is first line of defense against infection.*
4 High Risk for Infection *r.t. immature immune system, invasive procedures*	• Is free from nosocomial infections during hospitalization; is afebrile	• Assess and record VS q1-2h and prn • Separate the VLBW infant from other infants known to have infections; if possible, separate the nurse also • Maintain thermoneutral environment

NURSING DIAGNOSES	OUTCOME CRITERIA	INTERVENTIONS
		• Maintain strict hand-washing before and after patient contact; provide gloves for all patient contacts
		RATIONALE: *The VLBW infant has little resistance to infection due to immaturity of immune response and minimal antibody protection.*
5 Knowledge Deficit *r.t. lack of experience with care of immature infant*	• Parents verbalize concerns; discuss physiology of low birth weight treatment rationale; ask questions	• Listen, provide information - assess parents' level of anxiety and use of coping mechanisms - provide factual information about low birth weight; encourage questions - provide ongoing information about infant's progress
	• Parents perform holding, feeding, dressing, diapering, soothing, stimulating skills	• Demonstrate holding, feeding, soothing, dressing, diapering techniques; involve parents in caregiving as condition permits
	• Parents perform required care procedures	• Describe, demonstrate required care techniques
	• Parents list reportable s/s: weight loss or no gain, poor feeding, fever, dyspnea, lethargy, twitching, tremors	• Describe, provide list of s/s to report to physician
	• Parents express confidence in ability to manage at home; possess written follow-up appointments for well-child care	• Facilitate planning for home care - refer to community resources as needed - explain need for well-child care - verify possession of follow-up appointments
		RATIONALE: *Knowledgeable, competent parents can monitor, intervene, and care for their infant in developmentally appropriate ways.*

OTHER LESS COMMON NURSING DIAGNOSES: *Impaired Gas Exchange; High Risk for Fluid Volume Deficit; Sensory Perceptual Alterations; Decreased Cardiac Output; High Risk for Aspiration; Ineffective Airway Clearance; High Risk for Altered Parenting; Ineffective Infant Feeding Pattern; Inability to Sustain Spontaneous Ventilation*

ESSENTIAL DISCHARGE CRITERIA

- Maintains normal axillary temperature
- Tolerates activity with minimal fluctuation in HR, BP, muscle and tone
- Takes, retains 90% of feedings, gains weight
- Parents perform required care techniques and knowledge of s/s of complications to report to PCP

APPENDIXES

CONTENTS

APPENDIX A: ABBREVIATIONS

Abbreviations used in this book

ABG(s) arterial blood gas(es)
ABO blood groups A, B, and O
ADL(s) activities of daily living
AIDS acquired immunodeficiency syndrome
APIB assessment of preterm infant behavior
APPT activated partial thromboplastin time
AZT azidothymidine

Baso basophils
B.E. base excess
bid twice daily
BM(s) bowel movement(s)
BP blood pressure
bpm beats per minute
BPP biopshysical profile
BSC bedside commode
BUN blood urea nitrogen
BW birth weight

C centigrade
Ca calcium
cal calories
Ca:PO$_4$ calicum to phosphorous ratio
CBC complete blood count
C/DB cough, deep breathe
CDC communicable disease controls
CHF congestive heart failure
cm centimeter
CMV cytomegalovirus
CNS central nervous system
C.O. cardiac output
CO$_2$ carbon dioxide
CPK creatine phosphokinase
CPR cardiopulmonary resuscitation
CRT capillary refill time
C/S cesarean section
CVP central venous pressure

d day
DIC disseminated intravascular coagulation
dL deciliter
DTR deep tendon reflex

ECG electrocardiogram/graph
EEG electroencephalograph
EFM electronic fetal monitoring
ECG electrocardiogram/graph

ELISA enzyme-linked immunosorbent assays
Eos eosinophils
ET endotracheal
ETT endotracheal tube

F fahrenheit
FAS fetal alcohol syndrome
FHR fetal heart rate
FHT fetal heart tones
FOB foot of bed
FiO$_2$ fraction of inspired oxygen
FTT failure to thrive
FUO fever of undetermined origin

g gram
GA gestational age
GC gonorrhea
GFR glomerular filtration rate
GGT glutamyl transpeptidase
GI gastrointestinal

h hour
H&H hemoglobin and hematocrit
Hb hemoglobin
HbsAg surface antigen for hepatitis
Hct hematocrit
Hg mercury
HIV human immunodeficiency virus
HOB head of bed
hpf high power field
HR heart rate
HSV herpes simplex virus
H$_2$O water
H$_2$O$_2$ hydrogen peroxide

I&O intake and output
IDM infant of diabetic mother
IM intramuscular
IUGR intrauterine growth retardation
IUPC intracuterine pressure catheter
IV intravenous
IVIG intravenous gamma globulin

K potassium
kg kilogram

L liter
lab laboratory

LATCH latch, attack, nipple type, comfort, help with positioning infant (acronym for assessment)
lb pound
LDH lactic (acid) dehydrogenase
LGA large for gestational age
LOC level of consciousness

MCH mean corpuscular hemoglobin
MCHC mean corpuscular hemoglobin concentration
MCV mean corpuscular volume
mg milligram
MgSO$_4$ magnesium sulfate
min minute
mL milliliters
mm millimeters
mm^3 cubic millimeters
mmHg millimeters of mercury
MRI magnetic resonance imaging

Na sodium
ND nursing diagnosis
NEC necrotizing enterocolitis
NG nasogastric
NICU neonatal intensive care unit
NIDCAP neonatal individualized development care assessment program
NPH nasopharynx
NPO nothing by mouth
N/S normal saline
NST nonstress test
NTE neutral thermal therapy

O$_2$ oxygen
O$_2$ Hb oxygenated hemoglobin
O$_2$ sat oxygen saturation
OG orogastric
OPH oropharynx
OR operating room
oz ounces

P pulse
PA pulmonary artery
Pap Papanicolaou
PaCO$_2$ partial arterial pressure, carbon dioxide
PCO$_2$ partial arterial pressure, carbon dioxide
PCP primary care provider

PERL pupils equal and reactive to light
pH measure of acidity
PIH pregnancy induced hypertension
PIE pulmonary interstitial emphysema
PKU phenylketonuria
PMI point of maximum impact
PO, po orally, by mouth
PO_2 partial arterial pressure, oxygen
PO_4 phosphorous
PPHN persistent pulmonary hypertension
PR a specific interval on the ECG tracing
PRBC packed red blood cells
prn as needed
PT prothrombin time
PTL preterm labor
PTT partial thromboplastin time

QID four times daily
q every
qh every hour
qd every day
QRS a wave pattern on the ECG
qs quantity sufficient

RBC red blood cells
RDS respiratory distress syndrome
Rh rhesus antigen
ROM range of motion
RR respiratory rate
r.t. related to

SaO_2 saturated oxygen
sat saturation of oxygen
SBE subacute bacterial endocarditis
sec seconds
SGA small for gestational age
SGOT serum glutamic oxaloacetic transaminase
SGPT serum glutamic pyruvic transaminase
SIADH syndrome of inappropriate antidiuretic hormone
SIDS sudden infant death syndrome
SLE systemic lupus erythematosus
SOB shortness of breath
sp. gr. specific gravity
SPROM spontaneous preterm rupture of membranes
SQ subcutaneous
s/s signs and symptoms
STD sexually transmitted diseases
SW social work

TCDB turn, cough, deep breathe
TCM transcutaneous monitor
TCO_2 total carbon dioxide
TEF tracheoesophageal fistula
THb total hemoglobin
TID three times daily
TORCH test for toxoplasmosis, rubella, cytomegalic inclusion disease, and herpes simplex
TPR temperature, pulse, respirations
TPN total parenteral nutrition
TTN transient tachypnea of the newborn

UC uterine contractions
μg microgram
ung ointment
URI upper respiratory infection
UTI urinary tract infection

VDRL test for venereal disease
VLBW very low birth weight
VS vital signs

WBC white blood cells
wgt weight
WNL within normal limits

x times, frequency

ABBREVIATIONS

APPENDIX B: NORMAL VALUES (NEONATAL)

This appendix is organized in the way that test results are commonly grouped by laboratories.

SERUM ELECTROLYTES
SERUM CHEMISTRIES
COMPLETE BLOOD COUNT (CBC)
DIFFERENTIAL BLOOD COUNT
OTHER BLOOD STUDIES
URINE VALUES
CEREBROSPINAL FLUID
STOOL
OTHER
SWEAT
BLOOD GASES
VITAL SIGNS

SERUM ELECTROLYTES

TEST	SPECIMEN	AGE (preterm dependent on GA)	RANGE
Sodium (Na)	Serum	Preterm	133-148 mmol/L
		Newborn	130-145 mmol/L
Potassium (K)	Serum	Preterm	4.5-7.2 mmol/L
		Newborn	4.5-6.8 mmol/L
Chloride (Cl)	Serum	Preterm	100-117 mmol/L
		Newborn	95-110 mmol/L

SERUM CHEMISTRIES

TEST	SPECIMEN	AGE (preterm dependent on GA)		RANGE
Bicarbonate	Venous Arterial	Preterm		18-26 mmol/L
		Newborn		20-26 mmol/L
Bilirubin				
Total	Cord blood	0-1 d		< 2.0 mg/dL
	Serum	0-1 d		< 6.0 mg/dL
		1-2 d		< 8.0 mg/dL
		2-5 d		< 12.0 mg/dL
		> 5 d		2-1.0 mg/dL
Conjugated	Serum	Newborn		0-0.2 mg/dL
BUN	Serum	Preterm		3.1-25.5 mg/dL
		Newborn		6-30 mg/dL
Calcium, ionized (Ca)	Serum	Preterm		6-10 mg/dL
		Newborn	3-24 h	4.3-5.1 mg/dL
			24-48 h	4.0-4.7 mg/dL
Calcium, total	Serum	Newborn	3-24 h	9.0-10.6 mg/dL
			24-48 h	7.0-12.0 mg/dL
			4-7 d	9.0-10.9 mg/dL
Creatinine	Serum	Preterm		0.6-2.0 mg/dL
		Newborn		0.3-1.0 mg/dL
Creatinine Clearance (endogenous)	Serum	Newborn		40-65 mL/min/1.73 m^2
Glucose	Serum	Preterm		30-125 mg/dL
		Newborn	1 d	40-125 mg/dL
Glucose, 2 h pc	Serum	Preterm		40-125 mg/dL
		Newborn		< 120 mg/dL

Magnesium	Plasma	0-6 d	1.2-2.6 mg/dL
Protein, Total	Serum	Newborn	4.6-7.4 g/dL

COMPLETE BLOOD COUNT (CBC)

TEST	SPECIMEN	AGE (preterm dependent on GA)	RANGE
Erythrocyte count (RBC count)	Whole blood		Millions of cells/mm^3
		Preterm	4.0-4.4
		1-3 d (capillary)	4.0-6.6
Erythrocyte Sedimentation Rate (ESR)	Whole blood	Newborn	0-10 mm/h
Hb	Whole blood	Preterm	14.5-18.4 g/dL
		1-3 d (capillary)	14.5-22.5 g/dL
Hct *Percent PRBC (V Red Cells / V Whole Blood Cells x 100)*	Whole blood	Preterm	45-47%
		1 d (capillary)	48-69%
Platelet count (thrombocyte count)	Whole blood	Preterm	120-180 x $10^3/mm^3$
		Newborn	84-478 x $10^3/mm^3$
Reticulocyte count	Whole Blood	1 d	0.4-0.6%
		7 d	< 0.1-1.3%

DIFFERENTIAL BLOOD COUNT

TEST	SPECIMEN	AGE (preterm dependent on GA)	RANGE
Leukocyte differential	Whole Blood		
neutrophils—"bands"		Preterm	5-8%
		Newborn	3-5%
neutrophils—"segs"		Preterm	40-55%
		Newborn	54-62%
lymphocytes		Preterm	9-41%
		Newborn	25-33%
monocytes		Preterm	5-10%
		Newborn	3-7%
eosinophils		Preterm	2-3%
		Newborn	1-3%
basophils		Preterm	0-0.75%
		Newborn	0-0.75%

OTHER BLOOD STUDIES

TEST	SPECIMEN	AGE (preterm dependent on GA)	RANGE	
Bleeding time	Whole Blood	Newborn	2 min	
Clotting time	Whole Blood	Newborn	5-8 min	
Fibrinogen	Whole Blood	Newborn	0.18-0.38 g/dL	
PT	Whole Blood	Newborn	12-21 sec	
PTT	Whole Blood	Newborn	40-80 sec	
Immunoglobins, total	Whole Blood		1gG	1gM
		Preterm	186-728	2.1-39.4
		Newborn	69-352	5.5-432

URINE VALUES

TEST	SPECIMEN	AGE (preterm dependent on GA)	RANGE
Bilirubin	Urine	Preterm Newborn	negative negative
Creatinine	Urine	Newborn	10.4-19.7 mg/kg per 24h
Glucose	Urine	Preterm Newborn	negative negative
pH	Urine	Newborn/neonate	5-7 U
Occult blood	Urine	Preterm Newborn	negative negative
Osmolarity	Urine	Newborn	50-600 mOsm/L
Sp. Gr.	Urine	Preterm Newborn	1.001-1.020 U 1.006-1.018 U
Sediment: Casts: Hyaline seen occasionally (0-1) RBC WBC	Urine	Preterm	Not seen
		Newborn	Not seen
Cells:	Urine		
RBC		Newborn	0-2/hpf
WBC		Newborn, male Newborn, female	0-3/hpf 0-5/hpf
Epithelial		Newborn	Few
Bacterial			No organisms
Field Spun			< 20 organisms per hpf
Volume	Urine	Newborn	50-300 mL per 24h

CEREBROSPINAL FLUID

TEST	SPECIMEN	AGE (preterm dependent on GA)	RANGE
Cell count	CSF	Newborn	0-20 mononuclear cells per mL
			0-10 polymorphonuclear cells per mL
			0-800 RBC per mL
		Neonate	0-5 mononuclear cells per mL
			0-10 polymorphonuclear cells per mL
			0-50 RBC per mL
Pressure	CSF	Newborn	70-180 mm of water
Protein	CSF		
Total protein		Preterm	65-150 mg/dL
		Newborn	8-32 mg/dL

STOOL

TEST	SPECIMEN	AGE (preterm dependent on GA)	RANGE
Fat	Feces	Infant, breast-fed	< 1 g per 24h
Occult blood	Feces	Newborn	Negative

OTHER

TEST	SPECIMEN	AGE (preterm dependent on GA)	RANGE
Albumin	Plasma	Preterm	3.1-5.2 g/dL
		Full term < 6 d	2.5-3.4 g/dL
Pancreatic isoenzymes	Serum	Cord blood – 8 months	0-34%
Phosphatase, alkaline	Serum	26-27 weeks	320±87
		28-29 weeks	292±87
		30-31 weeks	281±85
		32-33 weeks	254±72
		34-35 weeks	236±62
		36 weeks	207±60
Phosphorus		Preterm	5.6-11.7 mg/dL
		Newborn	4.9-9.5 mg/dL
Theophylline		Newborn	5-10 µg/ml
Thyroxine			
Free (FT)			
Total (T)	Serum	Newborn (lower in VLBW)	11.5-24 µg/dL
		Neonate	9-18 µg/dL

NORMAL VALUES

SWEAT

TEST	SPECIMEN	AGE (preterm dependent on GA)	RANGE
Chloride	Sweat	Newborn	< 40 mmol/L
Sodium	Sweat	Newborn	< 40 mmol/L

BLOOD GASES

TEST	SPECIMEN	AGE (preterm dependent on GA)	RANGE
pH	Whole blood (arterial)	Preterm Full term birth 1 d	7.35-7.45 7.11-7.36 7.29-7.45
PO_2	Whole blood (arterial)	> 1 h of age 1 d	55-80 mmHg 54-95 mmHg
PCO_2	Whole blood (arterial)	Newborn	27-40 mmHg
Base excess	Whole blood	Newborn	(-2)-(-2) mmol/L
Oxygen saturation	Whole blood (arterial)	Newborn	87-97%
Bicarbonate	Whole Blood	Preterm Newborn	18-26 mmol/L 20-26 mmol/L

VITAL SIGNS

		FULL TERM	PRETERM *dependent on gestation and age
Blood pressure	systolic diastolic	60-80 mmHg 40-50 mmHg	*variable dependent on gestation and age
HR (apical)		110-160 bpm	120-160 bpm Fetus 110-180 bpm
Respiration		40-60 breaths per minute	40-60 breaths per minute
Temperature	axillary (skin)	35.5-37.5°C 97.6-98.4°F	Varies with GA, weight
	rectal (core)	36.5-37.0°C 96-99.5°F	

APPENDIX C: NORMAL VALUES (PERINATAL/MATERNAL)

This appendix is organized in the way that test results are commonly grouped by laboratories.

BLOOD	**DIFFERENTIAL BLOOD COUNT**	**BLOOD GASES**	**URINE (OUTPUT)**
HEMATOLOGY	**BLOOD COAGULATION**	**URINALYSIS**	**VITAL SIGNS**

BLOOD

TEST	REFERENCE RANGE
Albumin	3.0-5.0 g/dL
BUN	20-25 mg/dL
Calcium	8.5-10.5 mg/dL
Chloride	95-109 mEq/L
Cholesterol	110-300 mg/dL
CO_2	24-32 mEq/L
CPK	20-230 IU/L
Creatinine	0.7-1.4 mg/dL
Creatinine clearance	81-134 ml/min
GGT	3-60 IU/L
Glucose	65-140 mg/dL
Iron	65-120 μg/dL
LDH	100-225 IU/L
Potassium	3.5-5.2 mEq/L
SGOT	7-40 IU/L
SGPT	0-45 IU/L
Sodium	135-145 mEq/L
Total Protein	5.5-7.5 g/dL
Triglycerides	10-190 mg/dL
Valproic acid	Therapeutic 50-100 μg/mL

HEMATOLOGY

TEST	REFERENCE RANGE
Hb	10-14 g/dL
Hct	32-42%
MCH	29-32 pg
MCHC	30-36%
MCV	$82\text{-}96/u^3$
Platelet count	$150{,}000\text{-}350{,}000/mm^3$
RBC	$4\text{-}5.5\ M/mm^3$
WBC	$5\text{-}15\ kg/mm^3$

DIFFERENTIAL BLOOD COUNT

TEST	%	ABSOLUTE
Bands	0-11	< 10% of total differential
Baso	0-2	0-0.2
Eos	0-3	0-0.5
Left shift		RBC morph
Lymphs	21-45	1-4.8
Mono	2-9	0-0.8
Neutrophils	42-77	1.8-7.7
Reticulocytes	0.5-1.5	
Sed rate west	0-20	

BLOOD COAGULATION

TEST	REFERENCE RANGE
Bleeding time	1-3 (2-4) min
Coagulation time	6-10 min
D-Dimer	< 0.5 mg/dL
Fibrinogen	400 mg/dL
PT	12-14 sec
PTT	60-70 sec

BLOOD GASES

TEST	REFERENCE RANGE
B.E.	-2 to +2 mEq/L
CO Hb	0.0-9.0% (tHb)
O_2 ct	15-23 (Vol %)
O_2 Hb	94-100%
PCO_2	34-46 mmHg
pH	7.35-7.45
PO_2	75-100 mmHg
SaO_2	91.9-98.5%
T Hb	12.0-18.0 (G%)
TCO_2	23-27 mm/L

URINALYSIS

TEST	REFERENCE RANGE
Bacteria	0-2+
Bilirubin	negative
Blood	negative
Casts	cast per hpf
Clarity	clear
Color	amber
Crystals	present
Epithelial cells	few
Glucose	negative g/dL
Ketones	negative
Leukocyte esterase	negative
Mucus	few
pH	5-8 U
Protein	negative
RBC	0-2 # hpf
Sp. gr.	1.003-1.035 U
Urobilinogen	0-4 EU/24 h
WBC	0-4 # hpf

URINE

TEST	REFERENCE RANGE
Output	50-60 mL/h

VITAL SIGNS

TEST		REFERENCE RANGE
Temperature		
	core	36.5-37.6°C (97.7-99.7°F)
	oral	0.5°C (0.9°F) lower than rectal
	rectal	0.1°C (0.2-1.2°F) higher than oral
Pulse		70-90 bpm
Respiration		12-20 breaths per minute
BP		
	diastolic	60-80 mmHg
	systolic	95-120 mmHg

APPENDIX D: DEFINITIONS, CARE PLAN TOPICS

GENERAL

Education for Discharge: Teaching the parent/patient/family to perform care after discharge. Various situations are addressed in the subsections of this care plan.

ANTEPARTUM

Abruptio Placentae: Premature separation of the placenta occurring before the third stage of labor.

Cancer: The presence of cancer cells; in the antepartal period the cancer may be preexisting or experience rapid growth and initial diagnosis; a cellular tumor that invades and metastasizes; categories are carcinoma and sarcoma.

Cardiac Disease: An alteration in cardiac function due to congenital malformation or an active or historic disease process.

Chemical Dependency: Intermittent or chronic use of stimulants or depressants resulting in alterations in mental and physiological function.

Diabetes Mellitus: Diabetic mothers may be hospitalized during the last trimester of pregnancy to regulate insulin needs, which are usually higher than during the previous two trimesters, and to monitor fetal well-being because of the increased fetal and neonatal morbidity and mortality associated with maternal diabetes.

Domestic Violence: Physical and/or psychological abuse by an intimate partner; increases the risk of PTL in pregnant women.

Ectopic Pregnancy: Implantation of blastocyst in any place other than the uterine cavity, usually in the fallopian tube.

Genital/Vaginal Tract Infection: An infection in any part of the urinary tract, caused by bacteria, primarily *Escherichia coli*; risk and severity are increased by conditions such as urinary tract obstruction, urinary stasis, recent urethral instrumentation, and septicemia.

Herpes Simplex: A member of a family of large DNA viruses; can persist in a latent state; organism invades the sensory nerve endings. Risk of neonatal infection is estimated to be 5% in recurrent cases, higher in primary cases.

HIV/AIDS: AIDS includes the final stages of a wide range of health problems caused by the HIV type I. This virus attacks the cell-mediated immune system through invasion of T4 lymphocytes. The infected person becomes vulnerable to opportunistic infections and cancers.

Hyperemesis Gravidarum: Excessive or pernicious vomiting during pregnancy, potentially leading to dehydration after starvation.

Hypertension in Pregnancy (Preeclampsia, Toxemia): Syndrome of hypertension, edema, and proteinuria occurring during the second half of pregnancy, characteristically in primigravidas; resolves within 10 days postpartum; the etiology is unknown but could be caused by increased vasoconstrictor tone, abnormal prostaglandin action, or immunological factors.

Infectious Disorders: An invasion of one or more systems by bacteria or viral process(es).

Isoimmune Disease: Production of antibodies, usually by the mother, against a substance produced by the same species, such as Rh sensitization.

Multiple Gestation: A pregnancy that has more than one embryo/fetus.

Placenta Previa: Total, partial, or low implantation of the placenta over the internal cervical os; occurs most often in multiparas. Total and partial placenta previa prohibits vaginal delivery. With low implantation the fetus can sometimes be delivered vaginally with the presenting part acting as a tamponade against the placenta.

Preterm Labor: Physiological process by which the fetus is expelled from the uterus before the completion of 37 weeks of gestation.

Rupture of Membranes (Spontaneous Preterm): Rupture of the bag of waters 12 h or more before the onset of labor. The etiology is unknown but it is associated with hydramnios, multiple gestation, PTL, cervical incompetence, trauma, and amnionitis.

Thromboembolic Dysfunction: An abnormal vascular condition associated with thrombosis formation within a blood vessel, which develops as a result of stasis, hypercoagulability, or damage to the internal lining of the vein. This condition can occur in superficial or deep veins.

Urinary Tract Infection: An infection in any part of the urinary tract, caused by bacteria, primarily *Escherichia coli*; risk and severity are increased by urinary tract obstruction, urinary stasis, recent urethral instrumentation, and septicemia.

INTRAPARTUM

Labor Assessment and Support: The physiological process by which the fetus is expelled from the uterus. Early labor: dilation of 0 to 4 cm with mild to moderate irregular contractions. Active labor: dilation of 4 cm with moderate to strong regular contractions every 2 to 5 min. Transitional labor: dilation of 8 to 10 cm with strong contractions.

Dysfunctional Labor: Labor that falls outside of the normal labor curve; uncoordinated uterine contractions, failure of the cervix to dilate or presenting part to descend in the face of uterine contractions. Categorized as hypotonic or hypertonic uterine dysfunction.

Labor Induction/Augmentation: Oxytocin infusion may be used to either begin the labor process or to augment a labor that is progressing slowly because of inadequate uterine activity.

Prolapsed Umbilical Cord: Protrusion of the umbilical cord in advance of the presenting part. This should be suspected after amniotomy or spontaneous gross rupture of membranes and should be ruled out by vaginal examination.

Fetal Stress: A symptom complex indicative of a critical response to stress; may include hypoxia and/or acidosis.

Vaginal Delivery: The stage of expulsion of the fetus, placenta, and membranes from the mother at birth after complete dilation of the cervix.

Vaginal Recovery: The fourth stage of labor, the first hour postpartum.

Cesarean Delivery (pre-op): Delivery of a fetus through a uterine incision. Most common is the transverse lower uterine segment incision, with the classic vertical cesarean incision done less frequently.

POSTPARTUM

Breastfeeding: The provision of breast milk for infant nutrition at the breast.

Cesarean Delivery (post-op): Delivery of a fetus through a uterine incision. The most common incision is a transverse lower uterine segment incision; the classic vertical cesarean incision is done less frequently.

Early Discharge (Vaginal Delivery): Discharge from the delivery setting within a short time frame after vaginal delivery, usually 6 to 8 h.

Grief, Perinatal Loss: A natural human response to any loss, whether the loss is real, perceived, threatened, or anticipated.

Postpartum Hemorrhage: Post-delivery maternal bleeding resulting from uterine atony, lacerations, and/or retained products of conception. Predisposing factors include overdistended uterus, precipitous delivery, prolonged labor, chorioamnionitis, PIH/PTL treated with magnesium sulfate.

Thrombophlebitis: An abnormal vascular condition associated with thrombosis formation within a blood vessel, which develops as a result of stasis, hypercoagulability, or damage to the internal lining of the vein; can occur in superficial or deep veins.

Tuberculosis: A chronic, acute or subacute infectious disease caused by the tubercle bacillus, most commonly affecting the alveolar structure of the lung. Conical presentation varies from asymptomatic with only a positive skin test to extensive pulmonary and systemic involvement.

Vaginal Delivery (Postpartum): Care, after delivery of a fetus through the vaginal canal, throughout the maternal recovery period until hospital/birth center discharge.

NEWBORN

Circumcision: The removal of the foreskin (prepuce) covering the glans penis. This decision is made by parents based on cultural, religious, and/or personal beliefs.

Family Transition, Infant Integration: Interventions promoting bonding and attachment, and a method of assessing parent-infant interaction that helps to provide individualized, need-specific parent teaching and continuity of care.

Healthy Newborn: The transitional period after birth until discharge from the delivery setting.

Physiologic Jaundice: Elevation of unconjugated serum bilirubin concentration demonstrated by jaundice. Caused by hemolytic disorders, infection, enzymatic deficiencies, polycythemia maternal ingestion of sulfonamides or salicylates.

COMPROMISED NEONATE

Air Leak Syndrome: Collection of air or gas in the pleural space, causing the lung to collapse; may be partial or total collapse, open or communicating pneumothorax; occurs as a result of an open chest wound that permits entry of air.

Anemia: An RBC volume of 25 mL/kg, usually due to acute and/or chronic episodes of hemorrhage, RBC destruction, and blood sampling for laboratory analysis; neonates have a natural propensity toward physiologic anemia.

Apnea of Prematurity: Immature respiratory control mechanism and central responsiveness to carbon dioxide; may be associated with infection, impaired oxygenation, thermal instability, gastroesophageal reflux, metabolic derangement, drugs, or intracranial pathology.

Asphyxia: A clinical entity in which the fetus or newborn sustains an impairment in respiratory gas exchange. Perinatal asphyxia implies a combination of hypoxemia, hypercapnia, and circulatory insufficiency. Neonatal asphyxia implies inadequate ventilation, hypoxemia, respiratory and metabolic acidosis, cardiovascular deterioration, and CNS depression.

Assisted Ventilation: Artificial mechanical ventilation to treat various ventilatory problems.

Behavioral-Based Care: A framework for the provision of neonatal care based on behavioral observations, assessments, and plan of care that integrates the infant's behavioral cues to enhance developmental outcomes.

Bowel Obstruction: An obstruction of the small or large intestine or rectum; requires surgical repair and may have future implications for nutrition and/or elimination.

Chemical Addiction Withdrawal: The signs and symptoms of a neonate's withdrawal from chemical substances that were either transplacental or directly administered.

Chronic Lung Disease (Bronchopulmonary Dysplasia): Chronic lung condition with obstructive bronchiolitis, hyperinfiltration, and pulmonary fibrosis secondary to treatment for respiratory distress syndrome. Treatment includes high oxygen concentrations delivered by positive pressure ventilation.

Cleft Lip, Cleft Palate: A congenital malformation of the lip and/or palate. Lip may be malformed unilaterally or bilaterally. Malformation of palate may involve the hard or soft palate or both. Surgical repair occurs within the first two years of life.

Cocaine Exposure: Infants born to mothers who took cocaine during pregnancy; infants usually exhibit drug withdrawal behaviors and are at increased risk for SIDS.

Congenital Heart Defect: Congenital malformation of the heart and its proximate blood vessels; may be classified as cyanotic and acyanotic defects.

Congenital Hip Dysplasia: Hip instability, subluxation to complete dislocation.

Congestive Heart Failure: The blood supply to the body is insufficient to meet the metabolic requirements of the organs.

Feeding Dysfunction: An alteration in feeding pattern; may be due to immaturity, neurologic impairment, or congenital malformation.

Fetal Alcohol Syndrome: Dysmorphic characteristics, prenatal/postnatal growth deficiency, and CNS dysfunction due to maternal ingestion of alcohol during the pregnancy.

Gastroschesis/Omphalocele: A full-thickness defect in the abdominal wall through which the uncovered intestines protrude; requires surgical intervention.

Gastrostomy: An artificial opening in the stomach through the skin to facilitate decompression and feeding and to reduce reflux.

HIV/AIDS: AIDS includes the final stages of a wide range of health problems caused by the HIV type I. This virus attacks the cell-mediated immune system through invasion of T4 lymphocytes. The infected person becomes vulnerable to opportunistic infections and cancers. Neonates delivered of mothers with AIDS/HIV may present with HIV-related health problems.

Hydrocephalus: Excessive cerebrospinal fluid within the ventricular and subarachnoid spaces.

Hyperbilirubinemia: Increased levels of bilirubin in the blood; conjugated due to defective excretion by the liver; unconjugated due to excessive bilirubin production.

Hypocalcemia: Blood calcium below normal levels; characteristics include hyperreactive deep tendon reflexes and muscle/abdominal cramps.

Hypoglycemia: An abnormally low serum glucose level, usually 40 mg/dL or less, associated with SGA infants,LGA infants, IDMs, and interruption of glucose administration.

Infant of Diabetic Mother: Infant born to a mother experiencing diabetes during pregnancy; infants are at high risk for hypoglycemia, polycythemia, respiratory distress, and hyperbilirubinemia.

Infectious Disorders: Generalized infection in the newborn, often caused by antepartal or intrapartal asymptomatic maternal infection. Acquired postnatal infection is usually due to contact with personnel or contaminated equipment.

Intracranial Hemorrhage: Hemorrhage in the periventricular and/or intraventricular space; most commonly seen in preterm infants or infants weighing less than 1500 g.

Isoimmune Disease: Production of antibodies, usually by the mother, against a substance produced by the same species, such as Rh sensitization.

Large for Gestational Age: Weight greater than the ninetieth percentile for gestational age.

Meconium Aspiration Syndrome: Fetal hypoxia frequently causes relaxation of the anal sphincter, passage of meconium, and gasping respiratory efforts, resulting in meconium aspiration in the tracheobronchilar airways. Suspected in a meconium-stained neonate, postmature infant, or an infant large or small for gestational age.

Necrotizing Enterocolitis: Ischemia of the intestinal tract and invasion of the mucosa with enteric pathogens. It occurs most frequently in small and asphyxiated preterm infants, in those with Hirschsprung's disease, after exchange transfusion, or with an aggressive feeding schedule.

Patent Ductus Arteriosus: Persistence of blood flow through the fetal ductus arteriosus, between the aorta and the main pulmonary artery.

Persistent Pulmonary Hypertension: Pulmonary hypertension, right-to-left shunting through fetal channels away from the pulmonary vascular bed, and a structurally normal heart; associated with meconium aspiration syndrome, congenital diaphragmatic hernia, RDS, sepsis, hyperviscosity of the blood, or hypoglycemia.

Postoperative Care, Infant: General nursing care following surgical intervention.

Post-Term Infant: A neonate born after 42 weeks gestation.

Preoperative Care, Infant: General nursing care that prepares the child and family for surgery.

Respiratory Distress Syndrome: Condition of decreased pulmonary gas exchange producing retention of carbon dioxide usually resulting from deficiency of surfactant in immature lungs.

Seizure Disorder: Sudden and sometimes violent involuntary motor movements of a group of skeletal muscles; generally are transitory and often involve disturbances in consciousness as well as motor-sensory and/or autonomic function.

Skin Care: Special attention paid to the fragile, thin skin of preterm infants.

Small for Gestational Age: Weight less than the tenth percentile for gestational age.

Spina Bifida: A congenital defect in the spinal vertebrae resulting in motor and sensory dysfunction of the trunk and lower extremities below the level of deformity and accompanied by nonfunctional bowel and bladder sphincters. Malformed cord and roots are contained in a sac and covered by a thin vascular membrane.

Talipes (club foot): A congenital malformation of the foot and/or ankle.

Thermal Instability: Inability of neonate to control their temperature without excessive use of calories or system compromise.

Trachesophageal Fistula: A congenital anomaly usually consisting of esophageal atresia combined with a connection of the esophagus and trachea by way of a fistula.

Transient Tachypnea of the Newborn: Transient pulmonary edema; associated with cesarean delivery. Recovery usually occurs in 24-48 h.

Very Low Birth Weight Infant: Infant born at less than 1000 g, at high risk for multiple systems problems.

APPENDIX E: NANDA NURSING DIAGNOSES

This list represents the NANDA nursing diagnoses approved for clinical use and testing (1992).

Pattern 1: Exchanging

1.1.2.1.*	Altered +**Nutrition**: More than body requirements
1.1.2.2.	Altered **Nutrition**: Less than body requirements
1.1.2.3.	Altered **Nutrition**: Potential for more than body requirements
1.2.1.1.	High Risk for **Infection**
1.2.2.1.	High Risk for Altered **Body Temperature**
1.2.2.2.	Hypothermia
1.2.2.3.	Hyperthermia
1.2.2.4.	Ineffective **Thermoregulation**
1.2.3.1.	**Dysreflexia**
1.3.1.1.	**Constipation**
1.3.1.1.1.	Perceived **Constipation**
1.3.1.1.2.	Colonic **Constipation**
1.3.1.2.	**Diarrhea**
1.3.1.3.	**Bowel** Incontinence
1.3.2.	Altered **Urinary** Elimination
1.3.2.1.1.	Stress Incontinence **(Urinary)**
1.3.2.1.2.	Reflex Incontinence **(Urinary)**
1.3.2.1.3.	Urge Incontinence **(Urinary)**
1.3.2.1.4.	Functional Incontinence **(Urinary)**
1.3.2.1.5.	Total Incontinence **(Urinary)**
1.3.2.2.	**Urinary** Retention
1.4.1.1.	Altered **Tissue Perfusion** (Specify Type) (Renal, cerebral, cardiopulmonary, gastrointestinal, peripheral)
1.4.1.2.1.	**Fluid** Volume Excess
1.4.1.2.2.1.	**Fluid** Volume Deficit
1.4.1.2.2.2.	High Risk for **Fluid** Volume Deficit
1.4.2.1.	Decreased **Cardiac** Output
1.5.1.1.	Impaired **Gas** Exchange
1.5.1.2.	Ineffective **Airway** Clearance
1.5.1.3.1.	Inability to Sustain Spontaneous **Ventilation**
1.5.1.3.2.	Dysfunctional **Ventilatory** Weaning Response (DVWR)
1.6.1.	High Risk for **Injury**
1.6.1.1.	High Risk for **Suffocation**
1.6.1.2.	High Risk for **Poisoning**
1.6.1.3.	High Risk for **Trauma**
1.6.1.4.	High Risk for **Aspiration**
1.6.1.5	High Risk for **Disuse Syndrome**
1.6.2.	Altered **Protection**
1.6.2.1.	Impaired **Tissue Integrity**
1.6.2.1.1.	Altered **Oral** Mucous Membrane
1.6.2.1.2.1.	Impaired **Skin** Integrity
1.6.2.1.2.2.	High Risk for Impaired **Skin** Integrity

Pattern 2: Communicating

2.1.1.1.	Impaired Verbal **Communication**

Pattern 3: Relating

3.1.1.	Impaired **Social Interaction**
3.1.2.	**Social Isolation**
3.2.1.	Altered **Role** Performance
3.2.1.1.1.	Altered **Parenting**
3.2.1.1.2.	High Risk for Altered **Parenting**
3.2.1.2.1.	**Sexual** Dysfunction
3.2.2.	Altered **Family** Processes
3.2.2.1.	**Caregiver** Role Strain
3.2.2.2.	High Risk for **Caregiver** Role Strain
3.2.3.1.	**Parental** Role Conflict
3.3.	Altered **Sexuality** Patterns

Pattern 4: Valuing

4.1.1.	**Spiritual Distress** (Distress of the Human Spirit)

Pattern 5: Choosing

5.1.1.1.	Ineffective Individual **Coping**
5.1.1.1.1.	Impaired **Adjustment**
5.1.1.1.2.	Defensive **Coping**
5.1.1.1.3.	Ineffective **Denial**
5.1.2.1.1.	Ineffective Family **Coping**: Disabling
5.1.2.1.2.	Ineffective Family **Coping**: Compromised
5.1.2.2.	Family **Coping**: Potential for growth
5.2.1.	Ineffective Management of **Therapeutic** Regimen (Individuals)
5.2.1.1.	**Noncompliance** (Specify)
5.3.1.1	**Decisional** Conflict (Specify)
5.4.	**Health** Seeking Behaviors (Specify)

Pattern 6: Moving

6.1.1.1.	Impaired Physical **Mobility**
6.1.1.1.1.	High Risk for **Peripheral Neurovascular** Dysfunction
6.1.1.2.	**Activity** Intolerance
6.1.1.2.1.	**Fatigue**
6.1.1.3.	High Risk for **Activity** Intolerance
6.2.1.	**Sleep** Pattern Disturbance
6.3.1.1.	**Diversional** Activity Deficit
6.4.1.1.	Impaired **Home Maintenance** Management
6.4.2.	Altered **Health Maintenance**
6.5.1.	Feeding **Self-Care Deficit**
6.5.1.1.	Impaired **Swallowing**
6.5.1.2.	Ineffective **Breastfeeding**
6.5.1.2.1.	Interrupted **Breastfeeding**
6.5.1.3.	Effective **Breastfeeding**
6.5.1.4.	Ineffective **Infant** Feeding Pattern
6.5.2.	Bathing/Hygiene **Self-Care Deficit**
6.5.3.	Dressing/Grooming **Self-Care Deficit**
6.5.4.	Toileting **Self-Care Deficit**
6.6.	Altered **Growth** and Development
6.7.	**Relocation** Stress Syndrome

Pattern 7: Perceiving

7.1.1.	**Body Image** Disturbance
7.1.2.	**Self-Esteem** Disturbance
7.1.2.1.	Chronic Low **Self-Esteem**
7.1.2.2.	Situational Low **Self-Esteem**
7.1.3.	**Personal** Identity Disturbance
7.2.	**Sensory/Perceptual** Alterations (Specify): visual, auditory, kinesthetic, gustatory, tactile, olfactory
7.2.1.1.	**Unilateral** Neglect
7.3.1.	**Hopelessness**
7.3.2.	**Powerlessness**

Pattern 8: Knowing

8.1.1.	**Knowledge** Deficit (Specify)
8.3.	Altered **Thought** Processes
9.1.1.	**Pain**
9.1.1.1.	Chronic **Pain**
9.2.1.1.	Dysfunctional **Grieving**
9.2.1.2	Anticipatory **Grieving**
9.2.2.	High Risk for **Violence:** Self-directed or directed at others
9.2.2.1.	High Risk for **Self-Mutilation**
9.2.3.	**Post-Trauma** Response
9.2.3.1.	**Rape-Trauma** Syndrome
9.2.3.1.1.	**Rape-Trauma Syndrome**: Compound Reaction
9.2.3.1.2.	**Rape-Trauma Syndrome**: Silent Reaction
9.3.1.	**Anxiety**
9.3.2.	**Fear**

* Numbers refer to location in *NANDA Nursing Diagnoses: Definitions and Classifications 1992-1993.*

+ Bold type indicates alphabetical location in Appendix E.

APPENDIX F: DEFINITIONS, NURSING DIAGNOSES

This appendix includes only the definitions and defining characteristics of those nursing diagnoses that are used in this book.
Abridged from NANDA Nursing Diagnoses: Definitions and Classification, 1992

ACTIVITY INTOLERANCE A state in which an individual has insufficient physiological or psychological energy to endure or complete required or desired daily activities. **Defining Characteristics:** Verbal report of fatigue or weakness; abnormal heart rate or blood pressure response to activity; exertional discomfort or dyspnea; electrocardiographic changes reflecting arrhythmias or ischemia.

ACTIVITY INTOLERANCE, HIGH RISK FOR A state in which an individual is at risk of experiencing insufficient physiological or psychological energy to endure or complete required or desired daily activities. **Defining Characteristics:** *Presence of risk factors such as:* History of previous intolerance; deconditioned status; presence of circulatory/respiratory problems; inexperience with the activity.

AIRWAY CLEARANCE, INEFFECTIVE A state in which an individual is unable to clear secretions or obstructions from the respiratory tract to maintain airway patency. **Defining Characteristics:** Abnormal breath sounds (rales [crackles], rhonchi [wheezes]); changes in rate or depth of respiration; tachypnea; cough, effective/ineffective, with or without sputum, cyanosis; dyspnea.

ANXIETY A vague uneasy feeling whose source is often nonspecific or unknown to the individual. **Defining Characteristics: Subjective:** Increased tension; apprehension; painful and persistent increased helplessness; uncertainty; fearful; scared; regretful; overexcited; rattled; distressed; jittery; feelings of inadequacy; shakiness; fear of unspecific consequences; expressed concerns regarding change in life events; worried; anxious. **Objective:** Sympathetic stimulation–cardiovascular excitation, superficial vasoconstriction, pupil dilation; restlessness; insomnia; glancing about; poor eye contact; trembling/hand tremors; extraneous movement (foot shuffling, hand/arm movements); facial tension; voice quivering; focus "self"; increased wariness; increased perspiration.

ASPIRATION: HIGH RISK FOR The state in which an individual is at risk for entry of gastrointestinal secretions, oropharyngeal secretions, solids or fluids into tracheo-bronchial passages. **Defining Characteristics:** *Presence of risk factors such as:* Reduced level of consciousness; depressed cough and gag reflexes; presence of tracheostomy or endotracheal tube; incomplete lower esophageal sphincter; gastrointestinal tubes; tube feedings; medication administration; situations hindering elevation of upper body; increased intragastric pressure; increased gastric residual; decreased gastrointestinal motility; delayed gastric emptying; impaired swallowing; facial/oral/neck surgery or trauma; wired jaws.

BODY IMAGE DISTURBANCE Disruption in the way one perceives one's body image. **Defining Characteristics:** A or B must be present to justify the diagnosis of Body Image Disturbance. **A =** verbal response to actual or perceived change in structure and/or function. **B =** nonverbal response to actual or perceived change in structure and/or function. The following clinical manifestations may be used to validate the presence of A or B. *Objective:* Missing body part; actual change in structure and/or function; not looking at body part; not touching body part; hiding or overexposing body part (intentional or unintentional); trauma to nonfunctioning part; change in social involvement; change in ability to estimate spatial relationship of body to environment. *Subjective:* Verbalization of: change in lifestyle; fear of rejection or of reaction by others; focus on past strength, function, or appearance; negative feelings about body; feelings of helplessness, hopelessness, or powerlessness; preoccupations with change or loss; emphasis on remaining strengths, heightened achievement; extension of body boundary to incorporate environmental objects; personalization of part or loss by name; depersonalization of part or loss by impersonal pronouns; refusal to verify actual change.

BODY TEMPERATURE, ALTERED: HIGH RISK FOR The state in which the individual is at risk for failure to maintain body temperature within normal range. **Defining Characteristics:** *Presence of risk factors such as:* Extremes of age; extremes of weight; exposure to cold/cool or warm/hot environments; dehydration; inactivity or vigorous activity; medications causing vasoconstriction/vasodilation; altered metabolic rate; sedation; inappropriate clothing for environmental temperature; illness or trauma affecting temperature regulation.

BOWEL INCONTINENCE A state in which an individual experiences a change in normal bowel habits characterized by involuntary passage of stool.

BREASTFEEDING, EFFECTIVE (Potential for Enhanced): The state in which a mother-infant dyad/family exhibits adequate proficiency and satisfaction with breastfeeding process. **Defining Characteristics:** *Major:* Mother able to position infant at breast to promote a successful latch-on response; infant is content after feeding; regular and sustained suckling/swallowing at the breast; appropriate infant weight patterns for age; effective mother/infant communication patterns (infant cues, maternal interpretation and response). *Minor:* Signs and/or symptoms of oxytocin release (let down or milk ejection reflex); adequate infant elimination patterns for age; eagerness of infant to nurse; maternal verbalization of satisfaction with the breastfeeding process.

BREASTFEEDING, INEFFECTIVE The state in which a mother, infant, or child experiences dissatisfaction or difficulty with the breastfeeding process. **Defining Characteristics:** *Major:* Unsatisfactory breastfeeding process. *Minor:* Actual or perceived inadequate milk supply; infant inability to attach onto maternal breast correctly; resisting latching on; no observable signs of oxytocin release; observable signs of inadequate infant intake; nonsustained suckling at the breast; insufficient emptying of each breast per feeding; persistence of sore nipples beyond the first week of breastfeeding; insufficient opportunity for suckling at the breast; infant exhibiting fussiness and crying within the first hour after breastfeeding; unresponsive to other comfort measures; infant arching and crying at the breast.

BREASTFEEDING, INTERRUPTED A break in the continuity of the breastfeeding process as a result of inability or inadvisability to put baby to breast for feeding. **Defining Characteristics:** *Major:* Infant does not receive nourishment at the breast for some or all of feedings. *Minor:* Maternal desire to maintain lactation and provide (or eventually provide) her breast milk for her infant's nutritional needs; separation of mother and infant; lack of knowledge regarding expression and storage of breast milk.

BREATHING PATTERN, INEFFECTIVE The state in which an individual's inhalation and/or exhalation pattern does not enable adequate pulmonary inflation or emptying. **Defining Characteristics:** Dyspnea, shortness of breath, tachypnea, fremitus, abnormal arterial blood gas, cyanosis, cough, nasal flaring, respiratory depth changes, assumption of 3-point position, pursed-lip breathing/prolonged expiratory phase, increased anteroposterior diameter, use of accessory muscles, altered chest excursion.

CARDIAC OUTPUT, DECREASED A state in which the blood pumped by an individual's heart is sufficiently reduced so that it is inadequate to meet the needs of the body's tissues. **Defining Characteristics:** Variations in blood pressure readings, arrhythmias; fatigue; jugular vein distention; color changes, skin and mucous membranes; oliguria; decreased peripheral pulses; cold clammy skin; rales; dyspnea, orthopnea; restlessness. **Other Possible Characteristics:** Change in mental status; shortness of breath; syncope; vertigo; edema; cough; frothy sputum; gallop rhythm; weakness.

CAREGIVER ROLE STRAIN* A caregiver's difficulty in performing the family caregiver role. **Defining Characteristics:** *Caregiver reports:* Not having enough resources to provide the care needed; finding it hard to do specific caregiving activities; worry about such things as the care receiver's health and emotional state, having to put the care receiver in an institution, and who will care for the care receiver if something should happen to the caregiver; feeling that caregiving interferes with other important roles in their lives; feelings of loss because the care receiver is like a different person or, in the case of a child, that the care receiver was never the child the caregiver expected; family conflict around issues of providing care; feeling stress or nervousness in their relationship with the care receiver; feeling depressed.

CAREGIVER ROLE STRAIN: HIGH RISK FOR* A caregiver is vulnerable for feeling difficulty in performing the family caregiver role. **Risk Factors (Defining Characteristics):** *Pathophysiological*: Illness severity of the care receiver; addiction or co-dependency; premature birth/congenital defect; discharge of family member with significant home care needs; caregiver health impairment; unpredictable illness course or instability in the care receiver's health; caregiver is female; psychological or cognitive problems in care receiver. *Developmental*: Caregiver is not developmentally ready for caregiver role, e.g., a young adult needing to provide care for middle-aged parent; developmental delay or retardation of the care receiver or caregiver. *Psychological*: Marginal family adaptation or dysfunction prior to the caregiving situation; marginal caregiver's coping patterns; past history of poor relationship between caregiver and care receiver; caregiver is spouse; care receiver exhibits deviant, bizarre behavior. *Situational*: Presence of abuse or violence; presence of situational stressors such as significant loss, disaster or crisis, poverty or economic vulnerability; major life events, e.g., birth, hospitalization, leaving home, returning home, marriage, divorce, employment, retirement, death; duration of caregiving required; inadequate housing, transportation, equipment, or community services; family/caregiver isolation; lack of respite and recreation for caregiver; inexperience with caregiving; caregiver's competing role commitments; complexity/amount of caregiving tasks.

*80% of caregivers reports one of more defining characteristics.

COMMUNICATION, IMPAIRED: VERBAL The state in which an individual experiences a decreased or absent ability to use or understand language in human interaction **Defining Characteristics:** Unable to speak dominant language; speaks or verbalizes with difficulty; does not or cannot speak; stuttering; slurring; difficulty forming words or sentences; difficulty expressing thought verbally; inappropriate verbalization; dyspnea; disorientation.

CONSTIPATION A state in which an individual experiences a change in normal bowel habits characterized by a decrease in frequency and/or passage of hard, dry stools. **Defining Characteristics:** Decreased activity level; frequency less than usual pattern; hard, formed stools; palpable mass; reported feeling of pressure or fullness in rectum; straining at stool. **Other Possible Characteristics:** Abdominal pain; appetite impairment; back pain; headache; interference with daily living; use of laxatives.

COPING, FAMILY: POTENTIAL FOR GROWTH Effective management of adaptive tasks by family member involved with the client's health challenge, family member exhibits desire and readiness for enhanced health and growth in regard to self and in relation to the client. **Defining Characteristics:** Family member attempts to describe growth impact of crisis on his or her own values, priorities, goals, or relationships; family member is moving in direction of lifestyle that supports and monitors health and the maturational processes; audits and negotiates treatment programs; generally chooses experiences that optimize wellness; individual expresses interest in making contact on a one-to-one basis or on a mutual-aid group basis with another person who has experienced a similar situation.

COPING, INEFFECTIVE (INDIVIDUAL) Impairment of adaptive behaviors and problem-solving abilities of a person in meeting life's demands and roles. **Defining Characteristics:** Verbalization of inability to cope or inability to ask for help; inability to meet role expectations; inability to meet basic needs; inability to problem-solve; alteration in societal participation; destructive behavior toward self or others; inappropriate use of defense mechanisms; change in usual communication patterns; verbal manipulation; high illness rate; high rate of accidents.

DIARRHEA A state in which an individual experiences a change in normal bowel habits characterized by the frequent passage of loose, fluid, unformed stools. **Defining Characteristics:** Abdominal pain; cramping; increased frequency; increased frequency of bowel sounds; loose, liquid stools; urgency. **Other Possible Characteristics:** Change in color.

FAMILY PROCESSES, ALTERED The state in which a family that normally functions effectively experiences a dysfunction. **Defining Characteristics:** Family system unable to meet physical needs of its members; family system unable to meet emotional, security, or spiritual needs of its members; parents do not demonstrate respect for each other's views on childrearing practices; inability to express/accept wide range of feelings; inability to express/accept feelings of members; inability to relate to each other for mutual growth and maturation; uninvolved in community activities; inability to accept/receive help appropriately; rigidity in function and roles; family not demonstrating respect for individuality and autonomy of its members; family unable to adapt to change/deal with traumatic experience constructively; family failing to accomplish current/past developmental task; unhealthy family decision-making process; failure to send and receive clear messages; inappropriate boundary maintenance; inappropriate/poorly communicated family rules, rituals, symbols; unexamined family myths; inappropriate level and direction of energy.

FATIGUE An overwhelming sustained sense of exhaustion and decreased capacity for physical and mental work. **Defining Characteristics:** *Major:* Verbalization of an unremitting and/or overwhelming lack of energy; inability to maintain usual routines. *Minor:* Perceived need for additional energy to accomplish routine tasks; increase in physical complaints; emotionally labile or irritable; impaired ability to concentrate; decreased performance; lethargic or listless; disinterest in surroundings/introspection; decreased libido; accident prone.

FEAR Feeling of dread related to an identifiable source which the person validates. **Defining Characteristics:** Ability to identify object of fear.

FLUID VOLUME DEFICIT The state in which an individual experiences vascular, cellular, or intracellular dehydration. **Defining Characteristics:** Change in urine output; change in urine concentration; sudden weight loss or gain; decreased venous filling; hemoconcentration; change in serum sodium. **Other Possible Characteristics:** Hypotension; thirst; increased pulse rate; decreased skin turgor; decreased pulse volume/pressure; change in mental state; increased body temperature; dry skin; dry mucous membranes; weakness.

FLUID VOLUME DEFICIT: HIGH RISK FOR The state in which an individual is at risk of experiencing vascular, cellular, or intracellular dehydration. **Defining Characteristics:** *Presence of risk factors such as:* Extremes of age; extremes of weight; excessive losses through normal routes, e.g., diarrhea; loss of fluid through abnormal routes, e.g., indwelling tubes; deviations affecting access to or intake or absorption of fluids, e.g., physical immobility; factors influencing fluid needs, e.g., hypermetabolic state; knowledge deficiency related to fluid volume; medications, e.g., diuretics.

FLUID VOLUME EXCESS The state in which an individual experiences increased fluid retention and edema. **Defining Characteristics:** Edema; effusion; anasarca; weight gain; shortness of breath, orthopnea; intake greater than output; S/3 heart sound; pulmonary congestion (chest x-ray); abnormal breath sounds, rales (crackles); change in respiratory pattern; change in mental status; decreased hemoglobin and hematocrit; blood pressure changes; central venous pressure changes; pulmonary artery pressure changes; jugular vein distention; positive hepatojugular reflex; oliguria; specific gravity changes, azotemia, altered electrolytes; restlessness and anxiety.

GAS EXCHANGE, IMPAIRED The state in which the individual experiences a decreased passage of oxygen and/or carbon dioxide between the alveoli of the lungs and the vascular system. **Defining Characteristics:** Confusion; somnolence; restlessness; irritability; inability to move secretions; hypercapnea; hypoxia.

GRIEVING, ANTICIPATORY Potential loss of significant object*; expression of distress at potential loss; denial of potential loss; guilt; anger; sorrow; choked feelings; changes in eating habits; alterations in sleep patterns; alterations in activity level; altered libido; altered communication patterns.

GRIEVING, DYSFUNCTIONAL Verbal expression of distress at loss*; denial of loss; expression of guilt; expression of unresolved issues; anger; sadness; crying; difficulty in expressing loss; alteration in eating habits, sleep or dream patterns, activity level, libido; idealization of lost object; reliving of past experiences; interference with life functioning; developmental regression; labile affect; alterations in concentration and/or pursuits of tasks.

* Object loss is used in the broadest sense; objects may include people, possessions, a job, status, home, ideals, parts and processes of the body.

GROWTH AND DEVELOPMENT, ALTERED: The state in which an individual demonstrates deviations in norms from his/her age group. **Defining Characteristics:** *Major:* Delay or difficulty in performing skills (motor, social, or expressive) typical of age group; altered physical growth; inability to perform self-care or self-control activities appropriate for age. *Minor:* Flat affect; listlessness, decreased responses.

HEALTH MAINTENANCE, ALTERED Inability to identify, manage, and/or seek out help to maintain health. **Defining Characteristics:** Demonstrated lack of knowledge regarding basic health practices; demonstrated lack of adaptive behaviors to internal/external environmental changes; reported or observed inability to take responsibility for meeting basic health practices in any or all functional pattern areas; history of lack of health-seeking behavior; expressed interest in improving health behaviors; reported or observed lack of equipment; financial and/or other resources; reported or observed impairment of personal support systems.

HYPERTHERMIA A state in which an individual's body temperature is elevated above his/her normal range. **Defining Characteristics:** *Major:* Increase in body temperature above normal range. *Minor:* Flushed skin, warm to touch; increased respiratory rate; tachycardia; seizures/convulsions.

HYPOTHERMIA The state in which an individual's body temperature is reduced below normal range. **Defining Characteristics:** *Major:* Reduction in body temperature below normal range; shivering (mild); cool skin; pallor (moderate). *Minor:* Show capillary refill; tachycardia; cyanotic nail beds; hypertension; piloerection.

INFANT FEEDING PATTERN, INEFFECTIVE A state in which an infant demonstrates an impaired ability to suck or coordinate the suck and/or swallow response. **Defining Characteristics:** Inability to initiate or sustain an effective suck; inability to coordinate sucking, swallowing, and breathing.

INFECTION: HIGH RISK FOR The state in which an individual is at increased risk for being invaded by pathogenic organisms. **Defining Characteristics:** *Presence of risk factors such as:* Inadequate primary defenses (broken skin, traumatized tissue, decrease in ciliary action, stasis of body fluids, change in pH secretions, altered peristalsis); inadequate secondary defenses (decreased hemoglobin, leukopenia, suppressed inflammatory response) and immunosuppression; inadequate acquired immunity; tissue destruction and increased environmental exposure; chronic disease; invasive procedures; malnutrition; pharmaceutical agents; trauma; rupture of amniotic membranes; insufficient knowledge to avoid exposure to pathogens.

INJURY: HIGH RISK FOR A state in which the individual is at risk of injury as a result of environmental conditions interacting with the individual's adaptive and defensive resources. **Defining Characteristics:** *Presence of risk factors such as: Internal:* Biochemical, regulatory function (sensory dysfunction, integrative dysfunction, effector dysfunction, tissue hypoxia); malnutrition; autoimmune; abnormal blood profile (leukocytosis/leukopenia, altered clotting factors, thrombocytopenia, sickle cell, thalassemia, decreased hemoglobin); physical (broken skin, altered mobility); developmental age (physiological, psychosocial); psychological (affective, orientation). *External:* Biological (immunization level of community, microorganism); chemical (pollutants, poisons, drugs, pharmaceutical agents, alcohol, caffeine, nicotine, preservatives, cosmetics, and dyes); nutrients (vitamins, food types); physical (design, structure, and arrangement of community, building and/or equipment); mode of transport/transportation; people/provider (nosocomial agents, staffing patterns; cognitive, affective, and psychomotor factors).

KNOWLEDGE DEFICIT (SPECIFY) **Defining Characteristics:** Verbalization of problem; inaccurate follow-through of instruction; inaccurate performance of test; inappropriate or exaggerated behaviors, e.g., hysterical, hostile, agitated, apathetic.

MOBILITY, IMPAIRED PHYSICAL A state in which the individual experiences a limitation of ability for independent physical movement. **Defining Characteristics:** Inability to purposefully move within the physical environment, including bed mobility, transfer, and ambulation; reluctance to attempt movement; limited range of motion; decreased muscle strength, control, and/or mass; imposed restrictions of movement, including mechanical, medical protocol; impaired coordination.

+SUGGESTED FUNCTIONAL LEVEL CLASSIFICATION
0 = completely independent
1 = requires use of equipment or device
2 = requires help from another person, for assistance, supervision or teaching
3 = requires help from another person and equipment device
4 = dependent, does not participate in activity.
+Code adapted from E. Jones, et al. *Patient Classification for Long-Term Care: Users' Manual*, HEW, Publication No. HRA-74-3107, November 1974.

NUTRITION, ALTERED: LESS THAN BODY REQUIREMENTS The state in which an individual experiences an intake of nutrients insufficient to meet metabolic needs. **Defining Characteristics:** Loss of weight with or without adequate food intake; reported inadequate food intake less than RDA (recommended daily allowance); weakness of muscles required for swallowing or mastication; body weight 20% or more under ideal; reported or evident of lack of food; aversion to eating; lack of interest in food; reported altered taste sensation; satiety immediately after ingesting food; abdominal pain with or without pathology; sore, inflamed buccal cavity; capillary fragility; abdominal cramping; diarrhea and/or steatorrhea; hyperactive bowel sounds; perceived inability to ingest food; pale conjunctival and mucous membranes; poor muscle tone; excessive loss of hair; lack of information, misinformation.

NUTRITION, ALTERED: MORE THAN BODY REQUIREMENTS The state in which an individual is experiencing an intake of nutrients which exceeds metabolic needs. **Defining Characteristics:** Weight 10% over ideal for height and frame; weight 20%* over ideal for height and frame; triceps skin fold greater than 15 mm in men, 25 mm in women; sedentary activity level. Reported or observed dysfunctional eating pattern: pairing food with other activities; concentrating food intake at the end of day; eating in response to external cues such as time of day, social situation; eating in response to internal cues other than hunger, e.g., anxiety.

*Critical characteristic

PAIN (Acute) A state in which an individual experiences and reports the presence of severe discomfort or an uncomfortable sensation. **Defining Characteristics:** *Subjective:* Describes or communicates (verbal or coded) pain. *Objective:* Guarding behavior, protective; self-focusing; narrowed focus (altered time perception, withdrawal from social contact, impaired thought process); distraction behavior (moaning, crying, pacing, seeking out other people and/or activities, restlessness); facial mask of pain (eyes lack luster, "beaten look", fixed or scattered movement, grimace); alteration in muscle tone (may span from listless to rigid); autonomic responses not seen in chronic stable pain (diaphoresis, blood pressure and pulse change, pupillary dilation, increased or decreased respiratory rate).

PAIN, CHRONIC A state in which the individual experiences pain that continues for more than six months in duration. **Defining Characteristics:** *Major:* Verbal report or observed evidence of pain experienced for more than 6 months. *Minor:* Fear of reinjury; physical and social withdrawal; altered ability to continue previous activities; anorexia; weight changes; changes in sleep patterns; facial mask; guarded movement.

***PARENTING, ALTERED** The state in which a nurturing figure(s) experiences an inability to create an environment which promotes the optimum growth and development of another human being.+ **Defining Characteristics:** Abandonment; runaway; verbalizes lack of control child; incidence of physical and psychological trauma; lack of parental attachment behaviors; inappropriate visual, tactile, auditory stimulation; negative identification of infant/child's characteristics; negative attachment of meanings to infant/child's characteristics; constant verbalization of disappointment in gender or physical characteristics of the infant/child; verbalization of resentment toward the infant/child; verbalization of role inadequacy; inattentive to infant/child needs; verbal disgust at body functions of infant/child; noncompliance with health appointments for self and/or infant/child; inappropriate caretaking behavior (toilet training, sleep/rest, feeding); inappropriate or inconsistent discipline practices; frequent accidents; frequent illness; growth and development lag in the child; history of child abuse or abandonment by primary caretaker; verbalizes desire to have child call him/herself by first name versus traditional cultural tendencies; child receives care from multiple caretakers without consideration for the needs of the infant/child; compulsively seeking role approval from others.

***PARENTING, ALTERED: HIGH RISK FOR** The state in which a nurturing figure(s) is at risk to experience an inability to create an environment which promotes the optimum growth and development of another human being. **Defining Characteristics:** Presence of risk factors such as: Lack of parental attachment behaviors; inappropriate visual, tactile, auditory stimulation; negative identification or attachment of meanings of infant/child's characteristics; constant verbalization of disappointment in gender or physical characteristics of the infant/child; verbalization of resentment toward the infant/child; verbalization of role inadequacy; inattentive to infant/child's needs; verbal disgust at body functions of infant/child; noncompliance with health appointments for self and/or infant/child; inappropriate caretaking behaviors (toilet training, sleep/rest, feeding); inappropriate or inconsistent discipline practices; frequent accidents; frequent illness; growth and development lag in the child; history of child abuse or abandonment by primary caretaker; verbalizes desire to have child call him/herself by first name versus traditional cultural tendencies; child receives care from multiple caretakers without consideration for the needs of the infant/child; compulsively seeking role approval from others.

*It is important to state as a preface to parenting diagnoses that adjustment to parenting in general is a normal maturational process that elicits nursing behaviors of prevention of potential problems and health promotion

PROTECTION, ALTERED The state in which an individual experiences a decrease in the ability to guard the self from internal or external threats such as illness or injury. **Defining Characteristics:** *Major:* Deficient immunity; impaired healing; altered clotting; maladaptive stress response; neurosensory alteration. *Minor:* Chilling; perspiring; dyspnea; cough; itching; restlessness; insomnia; fatigue; anorexia; weakness; immobility; disorientation; pressure sores.

ROLE PERFORMANCE, ALTERED Disruption in the way one perceives one's role performance. **Defining Characteristics:** Change in self-perception of role; denial of role; change in other's perception of role; conflict in roles; change in physical capacity to resume role; lack of knowledge of role; change in usual patterns of responsibility.

SELF-ESTEEM DISTURBANCE Negative self-evaluation of capabilities, or negative feelings about self or own capabilities, which may be directly or indirectly expressed. **Defining Characteristics:** Self-negating verbalizations; expressions of shame/guilt; evaluates self as unable to deal with events; rationalizes away/rejects positive feedback and exaggerates negative feedback about self; hesitant to try new things/situations; denial of problems obvious to others; projection of blame/responsibility for problems; rationalizing personal failures; hypersensitive to slight or criticism; grandiosity.

SENSORY/PERCEPTUAL ALTERATIONS: VISUAL, AUDITORY, KINESTHETIC, GUSTATORY, TACTILE, OLFACTORY (SPECIFY) A state in which an individual experiences a change in the amount or patterning of oncoming stimuli accompanied by a diminished, exaggerated, distorted, or impaired response to such stimuli. **Defining Characteristics:** Disoriented in time, in place, or with persons; altered abstraction; altered conceptualization; change in problem-solving abilities; reported or measured change in sensory acuity; change in behavior pattern; anxiety; apathy; change in usual response to stimuli; indication of body-image alteration; restlessness; irritability; altered communication patterns. **Other Possible Characteristics:** Complaints of fatigue; alteration in posture; change in muscular tension; inappropriate responses; hallucinations.

SEXUALITY PATTERNS, ALTERED The state in which an individual expresses concern regarding his/her sexuality. **Defining Characteristics:** *Major:* Reported difficulties, limitations, or changes in sexual behaviors or activities.

SKIN INTEGRITY, IMPAIRED A state in which the individual's skin is adversely altered. **Defining Characteristics:** Disruption of skin surface; destruction of skin layers; invasion of body structures.

SKIN INTEGRITY, IMPAIRED: HIGH RISK FOR A state in which the individual's skin is at risk of being adversely altered. **Defining Characteristics:** *Presence of risk factors such as: External (environmental):* Hypo- or hyperthermia; chemical substance; mechanical factors (shearing forces, pressure, restraint); radiation; physical immobilization; excretions/secretions; humidity. *Internal (somatic):* Medication; alterations in nutritional state (obesity, emaciation); altered metabolic state; altered circulation; altered sensation; altered pigmentation; skeletal prominence; developmental factors; alterations in skin turgor (change in elasticity); psychogenic; immunologic.

SLEEP PATTERN DISTURBANCE Disruption of sleep time causes discomfort or interferes with desired lifestyle. **Defining Characteristics:** Verbal complaints of difficulty falling asleep; awakening earlier or later than desired; interrupted sleep; verbal complaints of not feeling well-rested; changes in behavior and performance (increasing irritability, restlessness, disorientation, lethargy, listlessness); physical signs (mild fleeting nystagmus, slight hand tremor, ptosis of eyelid, expressionless face, dark circles under eyes, frequent yawning, changes in posture); thick speech with mispronunciation and incorrect words.

SOCIAL ISOLATION Aloneness experienced by the individual and perceived as imposed by others and as a negative or threatened state. **Defining Characteristics:** *Objective:* Absence of family, friends, or other supportive significant other(s); sad, dull affect; inappropriate or immature interests/activities for development age/stage; uncommunicative, withdrawn, no eye contact; preoccupation with own thoughts, repetitive, meaningless actions; projects hostility in voice, behavior; seeks to be alone or to exist in subculture; shows behavior unaccepted by dominant cultural group; evidence of physical/mental handicap or altered state of wellness. *Subjective:* Expresses feelings of aloneness imposed by others; expresses feelings of rejection; experiences feelings of difference from others; lacks significant purpose in life; unable to meet expectations of others; shows insecurity in public; expresses values acceptable to the subculture but unacceptable to the dominant cultural group; expresses interests inappropriate to developmental age/state.

SWALLOWING, IMPAIRED The state in which an individual has decreased ability to voluntarily pass fluids and/or solids from the mouth to the stomach. **Defining Characteristics:** *Major:* Observed evidence of difficulty in swallowing, e.g., stasis of food in oral cavity, coughing/choking. *Minor:* Evidence of aspiration.

THERMOREGULATION, INEFFECTIVE The state in which the individual's temperature fluctuates between hypothermia and hyperthermia. **Defining Characteristics:** Fluctuations in body temperature above or below the normal range. See also characteristics present in hypothermia and hyperthermia.

TISSUE INTEGRITY, IMPAIRED A state in which an individual experiences damage to mucous membrane and corneal, integumentary, or subcutaneous tissue. **Defining Characteristics:** *Major:* Damaged or destroyed tissue (cornea, mucous membrane, integumentary, or subcutaneous).

TISSUE PERFUSION, ALTERED: RENAL, CEREBRAL, CARDIOPULMONARY, GASTROINTESTINAL, PERIPHERAL (SPECIFY TYPE) The state in which an individual experiences a decrease in nutrition and oxygenation at the cellular level due to a deficit in capillary blood supply. **Defining Characteristics:** Skin temperature: cold in extremities. Skin color: dependent, blue or purple and pale on elevation; color does not return on lowering of leg; diminished arterial pulsations. Skin quality: shining; lack of lanugo; slow healing of lesions; gangrene; slow-growing, dry, brittle nails. Other: claudication; blood pressure changes in extremities; bruits.

URINARY ELIMINATION, ALTERED The state in which the individual experiences a disturbance in urine elimination. **Defining Characteristics:** Dysuria; frequency; hesitancy; incontinence; nocturia; retention; urgency.

URINARY RETENTION The state in which the individual experiences incomplete emptying of the bladder. **Defining Characteristics:** *Major:* Bladder distention; small, frequent voiding or absence of urine output. *Minor:* Sensation of bladder fullness; dribbling; residual urine; dysuria; overflow incontinence.

BIBLIOGRAPHY

Ackley, B., and G. Ladwig: *Nursing Diagnosis Handbook: A Guide to Planning Care*, Mosby Year Book, St. Louis, 1993.

Alfaro, Rosalinda: *Applications of Nursing Process: A Step-by-Step Guide*, J. B. Lippincott Company, Philadelphia, 1986.

Angelin, D., and R. Gibes: "Substance Abuse and Environmental Toxins," *Journal of Perinatal and Neonatal Nursing*, 1990, pp. 13-33.

Axton, Sharon E., and Terry Fugate: *Neonatal and Pediatric Critical Care Plans*, Williams and Wilkins Publishing Company, Baltimore, 1989.

_______: *Pediatric Care Plans*, Addison-Wesley Nursing, Redwood City, Calif., 1993.

Barnes, L. P.: "Tuberculosis: Implications for Patient Teaching," *MCN 18*, 1993, p. 224.

"The Battered Woman," *American College of Obstetricians and Gynecologists Technical Bulletin 124*, 1989, pp. 1-8.

Bays, J.: "The Care of Alcohol- and Drug-Affected Infants," *Pediatric Annals*, August 1992, pp. 485-495.

Beachy, P., and J. Deacon (Eds.): *Core Curriculum for Neonatal Intensive Care Nursing*, W. B. Saunders Company, Philadelphia, 1993.

Bellack, J. P., and P. A. Bamford: *Nursing Assessment: A Multidimensional Approach*, Jones and Bartlett Publishers, Boston, 1987.

Blackburn, Susan T., and Donna L. Loper: *Maternal, Fetal, and Neonatal Physiology: A Clinical Perspective*, W. B. Saunders, Philadelphia, 1992.

Bobak, Irene M., and Margaret D. Jensen: *Essentials of Maternity Nursing*, 3d ed, Philadelphia, Mosby Year Book, 1991.

_______ and _______: *Maternity and Gynecologic Care: The Nurse and the Family*, 5th ed., Mosby Year Book, St. Louis, 1993.

Boyd, M. W., and B. L. Tower: *Medical Surgical Nursing: A Study and Learning Tool*, Springhouse Corporation, Springhouse, Pa., 1988.

Buckley, Kathy, and Nancy W. Kulb: *High Risk Maternity Nursing*, 2d ed., Williams and Wilkins Publishing Company, Baltimore, 1992.

_______: *High Risk Maternity Nursing Manual*, Williams and Wilkins Publishing Company, Baltimore, 1990.

Bulechek, Gloria M., and Joanne E. McCloskey: *The Nursing Clinics of North America*, W. B. Saunders, Philadelphia, 1992.

_______: *Nursing Interventions: Treatments for Nursing Diagnoses*, W. B. Saunders, Philadelphia, 1985.

_______: *Nursing Interventions Classification (NIC): Iowa Intervention Project*, C. V. Mosby, St. Louis, 1992.

Carpenito, Lynda Juall: *Handbook of Nursing Diagnosis,* J. B. Lippincott Company, Philadelphia, 1987.

_______: *Handbook of Nursing Diagnosis,* 5th ed., J. B. Lippincott Company, Philadelphia, 1993.

_______: *Nursing Care Plans and Documentation*, J. B. Lippincott Company, Philadelphia, 1991.

_______: *Nursing Diagnosis: Application to Clinical Practice*, 5th ed., J. B. Lippincott Company, Philadelphia, 1993.

_______: *Nursing Diagnosis: Application to Clinical Practice*, 4th ed., J. B. Lippincott Company, Philadelphia, 1992.

_______: *Nursing Diagnosis: Application to Clinical Practice*, 3d ed., J. B. Lippincott Company, Philadelphia, 1989.

Carroll-Johnson, Rose Mary (Ed.) *North American Nursing Diagnosis Association Classification of Nursing Diagnoses: Proceedings of the Ninth Conference,* J. B. Lippincott Company, Philadelphia, 1991.

Centers for Disease Control: *Core Curriculum on Tuberculosis*, American Lung Association, New York, 1990.

Cohen, Susan M., and Andrea Hollingsworth: *Maternal, Neonatal, and Women's Health Nursing*, Springhouse Corporation, Springhouse, Pa., 1991.

_______, Carol A. Kenner, and Andrea O. Hollingsworth: *Maternal, Neonatal, and Women's Health Nursing*, Springhouse Corporation, Springhouse, Pa., 1992.

Cox, H., M. Hinz, M. S. Lubano, S. Newfield, N. Rindenour, M. Slater, and K. Sridaromont: *Clinical Application of Nursing Diagnosis: Adult, Child, Women's, Psychiatric, Terontic and Home Health Considerations*, 2d ed., F. A. Davis Company, Philadelphia, 1993.

Craft, Martha J., and Janice A. Denehy: *Nursing Interventions for Infants and Children*, W. B. Saunders, Philadelphia, 1990.

Creighton, Neal M., P. Feltz-Cohen, and J. Reighley: *Nursing Care Planning Guides, Set 6*, Williams and Wilkins Publishing Company, Baltimore, 1986.

Cvetkovich, T. A., and L. M. Frankel: "Current Management of HIV Infection in Children," *Pediatric Annals 22*(7), July 1993, pp. 428-434.

Deglin, J., and A. Vallerand: *Davis's Drug Guide for Nurses,* 3d ed., F. A. Davis Company, Philadelphia, 1993.

Dickason, E. J., M. O. Shult, and B. L. Silverman: *Maternal-Infant Nursing Care*, C. V. Mosby, St. Louis, 1990.

Dixon, S., K. Bresnahan, and B. Zukerman: "Cocaine Babies: Meeting the Challenge of Management," *Contemporary Pediatrics*, 1990, pp. 70-90.

Doenges, M. S., and M. F. Moorhouse: *Nurses' Pocket Guide: Nursing Diagnoses with Interventions*, F. A. Davis Company, Philadelphia, 1993.

"Downtime Final Report Form," Oregon Medical Laboratories, Eugene, Oregon, n.d.

Foster, R., M. Hunsburger, and J. Anderson: *Family Centered Nursing Care of Children*, W. B. Saunders Company, Philadelphia, 1989.

Freij, Bishara J., and John L. Sever: "Infectious Complications of Pregnancy," *Clinics in Perinatology 15*(2), 1988, pp. 163-181.

Gabbe, S., J. Neibyl, and J. Simpson: *Obstetrics: Normal and Problem Pregnancies*, 2d ed., Churchill Livingstone, New York, 1991.

Gordon, Marjory: *Manual of Nursing Diagnosis, 1993-1994*, Mosby Year Book, St. Louis, 1993.

Gosse, G.: "Neonatal Abstinence Syndrome," *The Canadian Nurse*, May 1992, pp. 17-22.

Greenberg, Cindy Smith (Ed.): *Nursing Care Planning Guides for Children*, Williams and Wilkins Publishing Company, Baltimore, 1989.

Gulanick, Meg R., Michele K. Puzas, and Cynthia R. Wilson: *Nursing Care Plans*

BIBLIOGRAPHY

for Newborns and Children, C. V. Mosby, St. Louis, 1992.

Gunderson, L. P., and C. Kenner (Eds.): *Care of the 24-25 Week Gestational Age Infant (Small Baby Protocol)*, Neonatal Network, Petaluma, Calif, 1990.

_______ and _______: *Handbook of Medical-Surgical Nursing*, Springhouse Corporation, Springhouse, Pa., 1994.

Hanson-Smith, B.: *Nursing Care Planning Guides for Childbearing Families*, Williams and Wilkins Publishing Company, Baltimore, 1989.

Hausman, Kathy A.: "Neurological Crises," in K. Vestal and C. A. Mckenzie (Eds.), *High Risk Perinatal Nursing*, C. V. Mosby, Philadelphia, 1983.

Henrikson, M., G. Wall, D. Lethbridge, and V. McClurg: "Nursing Diagnosis and Obstetric, Gynecologic, and Neonatal Nursing: Breastfeeding as an Example," *Journal of Obstetric, Gynecologic, and Neonatal Nurses 21*(6), pp. 446-456.

Holloway, Nancy M.: *Critical-Care Care Plans*, Springhouse Corporation, Springhouse, Pa., 1989.

Honn, A. W.: *A. W. Honn's Clinical Issues in Perinatal and Women's Health*, vol. 4, no. 2, J. B. Lippincott Company, Philadelphia, 1993.

Jaffe, Marie S., and Kathryn A. Melson: *Maternal Infant Health Care Plans*, Springhouse Corporation, Springhouse, Pa., 1989.

James, Susan Rowen, Sandra R. Mott: *Child Health Nursing: Essential Care of Children and Families*, Reading, Mass., Addison-Wesley Publishing, 1988.

Johnson, Suzanne Hall: *Nursing Assessment and Strategies for the Family at Risk*, J. B. Lippincott Company, Philadelphia, 1986.

Kenner, Carole, Ann Brueggemeyer, and Laurie P. Gunderson (Eds.): *Comprehensive Neonatal Nursing: A Physiologic Perspective*, W. B. Saunders Company, Philadelphia, 1993.

Kim, M., G. McFarland, and A. McLane: *Pocket Guide to Nursing Diagnoses*, 5th ed., C. V. Mosby, St. Louis, 1993.

Klaus, M. H., and A. A. Fanaroff: *Care of the High-Risk Neonate*, W. B. Saunders Company, Philadelphia, 1993.

Korones, S.: *High-Risk Newborn Infants: The Basis for Nursing Care*, 4th ed., C. V. Mosby, St. Louis, 1986.

Korones, Sheldon B., and Henrietta S. Bada-Elizey: *Neonatal Decision Making*, Mosby Year Book, St. Louis, 1993.

Ladewig, P., M. London, and S. Olds: *Essentials of Maternal-Newborn Nursing*, 2d ed., Addison-Wesley Nursing, Redwood City, Calif., 1990.

LeBlanc, K. B., and F. E. Foustell: "Assessment of the Neonatal Respiratory System," *AACN Clinical Issues in Critical Care Nursing 1*(2), 1990, pp. 401-408.

Lederer, J., G. Marculescu, B. Mosnik, and N. Seaby, *Care Planning Pocket Guide: A Nursing Diagnosis Approach,* Addison-Wesley, Redwood City, Calif., 1991.

Long, B. C., and W. J. Phipps: *Medical-Surgical Nursing*, C. V. Mosby, St. Louis, 1989.

_______ and V. L. Cassmeyer: *Medical-Surgical Nursing: A Nursing Process Approach*, 3d ed., C. V. Mosby, St. Louis, 1993.

Malinowski, J. S., C. G. Pedigo, and C. R. Phillips: *(1989) Nursing Care During the Labor Process*, 3d ed., F. A. Davis Company, Philadelphia, 1989.

Mandeville, L., and N. Troiamo: *High-Risk Intrapartum Nursing*, J. B. Lippincott Company, Philadelphia, 1992.

Marlow, Dorothy R., and Barbara A. Redding: *Textbook of Pediatric Nursing*, 6th ed., W.B. Saunders Company, Philadelphia, 1988.

Martin, Jean E.: *Intrapartum Management Modules*, Williams and Wilkins Publishing Company, Baltimore, 1990.

Martin, L., and S. Reeder: *Essentials of Maternity Nursing*, J. B. Lippincott Company, Philadelphia, 1991.

Martin, T., M. Cannobbio, E. Vargo Pacquette, and M. Fyfe Wells: *Patient Care Standards: Nursing Process, Diagnosis, Outcome*, 5th ed., Mosby Year Book, Baltimore, 1992.

Mattson, Susan, and Judy E. Smith: *Core Curriculum for Maternal-Newborn Nursing*, W. B. Saunders, Philadelphia, 1993.

May, K. A., and L. R. Mahlmeister: *Comprehensive Maternity Nursing*, J. B. Lippincott Company, Philadelphia, 1990.

Mayers, Marlene: *Clinical Care Plans: Pediatric Nursing*, Markham-McKenzie Publishers, Eugene, Oregon, 1993.

_______: *Clinical Care Plans: Perinatal Nursing*, Markham-McKenzie Publishers, Eugene, Oregon, 1991.

_______: *Clinical Care Plans: Orthopedic and Neurologic Nursing*, Markham-McKenzie Publishers, Eugene, Oregon, 1991.

McCloskey, J. C., and G. M. Bulechek: *Nursing Interventions Classification (NIC)*, Mosby Year Book, St. Louis, 1992.

Mercer, Ramona: *Parents at Risk*, Springer Publishing Company, New York, 1990.

Merenstein, Gerald, and Sandra L. Gardner: *Handbook of Neonatal Intensive Care*, 2d ed., C. V. Mosby, St. Louis, 1989.

Mott, S. R., S. R. James, and A. M. Sperhac: *Nursing Care of Children and Families*, 2d ed., Addison-Wesley Nursing, Redwood City, Calif., 1990.

NAACOG: *OGN Nursing Practice Resource: Neonatal Skin Care*, NAACOG, Washington, D.C., January 1992.

_______: *Standards for the Nursing Care of Women and Newborns*, 4th ed., NAACOG, Washington, D.C., 1991.

Nelson, N. P., and J. Beckel (Eds.): *Nursing Care Plans for the Pediatric Patient*, C. V. Mosby, St. Louis, 1987.

Newberger, Eli H.: *Child Abuse*, Little, Brown, and Company, Boston, 1982.

Noel, Nancy L., and Marylou Yam: "Domestic Violence: The Pregnant Battered Woman," *Nursing Clinics of North America 27*(4), 1992, pp. 871-884.

North American Nursing Diagnosis Association: *NANDA Nursing Diagnoses: Definitions and Classifications, 1992;* North American Nursing Diagnosis Association, Philadelphia, 1992.

_______: *Taxonomy with Complete Diagnoses*, North American Nursing Diagnosis Association, St. Louis, 1987.

_______: *Taxonomy I Revised 1990 with Official Nursing Diagnoses*, North American Nursing Diagnosis Association, St. Louis, 1990.

Nugent, Jan (Ed.): *Acute Respiratory Care of the Neonate*, NICU Incorporated, Petaluma, Calif., 1991.

Olds, Sally B., Marcia L. London, and Patricia W. Ludwig: *Maternal-Newborn Nursing*, 3d ed., Addison-Wesley Nursing, Menlo Park, Calif., 1988.

_______: *Maternal-Newborn Nursing: A Family Centered Approach*, 4th ed., Addison-Wesley Nursing, Redwood City, Calif., 1992.

Parker, Barbara, and Judith McFarlane: "Identifying and Helping Battered Pregnant Women," *MCN 16*, 1991, pp. 161-164.

Pillitteri, Adele: *Maternal and Child Health Nursing: Care of the Childbearing and Childrearing Family*, J. B. Lippincott Company, Philadelphia, 1992.

Rawlins, R., and P. Heacock: *Clinical Manual of Psychiatric Nursing*, 2d ed., Mosby Year Book, St. Louis, 1993.

Reeder, S. J., L. L. Martin, and D. Koniak: *Maternity Nursing*, J. B. Lippincott Company, Philadelphia, 1992.

_______, L. Mastroianmi, and L. Martin: *Maternity Nursing*, J. B. Lippincott Company, Philadelphia, 1990.

Samuelson, Julie J., Jill Foltz, and Martha J. Foxall: *Stress and Coping in Families of Children with Myelomeningocele*, W. B. Saunders, Philadelphia, 1992.

Schafer, Patricia, M. Kathleen Kelly, Karen Lehr, and Jacqueline Saracco: *Nursing Care Plans for the Child: A Nursing Diagnosis Approach*, Appleton & Lange, East Norwalk, Conn., 1988.

"Scoring Guidelines", *1994 Accreditation Manual for Hospitals, Vol III:* The Joint Commission on the Accreditatation of Health Care Organizations, Oakbrook Terrace, Il, 1993, p. 5.

Scott, G. B.: *Pediatric Immunity and Infectious Diseases*, Paper presented at NANN, 9th National Meeting, Orlando, Florida, September 8-12, 1993.

Segen, J.C.: *The Dictionary of Modern Medicine*, Parthenon Publishing Group, Park Ridge, New Jersey, 1992.

Servonsky, J., and S. R. Opas: *Nursing Management of Children*, Jones and Bartlett Publishers, Boston, 1987.

Sherwin, Laurie N., Mary Ann Acolovana, and Carol Toussle Weingarter: *Nursing Care of the Childbearing Family*, Appleton and Lange, East Norwalk, Conn., 1991.

Smith, D.: *Recognizable Patterns of Human Malformation*, 3d ed., W. B. Saunders, Philadelphia, 1982.

Sparks, Sheila M., and Cynthia M. Taylor: *Nursing Diagnosis Reference Manual*, 2d ed., Springhouse Corporation, Springhouse, Pa., 1993.

Speer, Kathleen Morgan: *Pediatric Care Plans*, Springhouse Corporation, Springhouse, Pa., 1990.

Task Force on Pediatric AIDS: "Pediatric Guidelines for Infection Control of Human Immunodeficiency Virus (Acquired Immunodeficiency Virus) in Hospitals, Medical Offices, Schools and Other Settings," *Pediatrics 82*(5), November 1988, n.p.

Thompson, June M., Gertrude K. McFarland, Jane E. Hirsch, and Susan M. Tucker: *Mosby's Clinical Nursing*, 3rd ed., St. Louis, Mosby, 1993.

Torrance, C., and K. Horns: "Appraisal and Caregiving for the Drug-Addicted Infant," *Neonatal Network 8*(3), 1989, pp. 49-59.

Tucker, Susan, and et al.: *Patient Care Standards: Nursing Process, Diagnosis, and Outcome*, 5th ed., Mosby Year Book, St. Louis, 1992.

Vallejo, J. G., and J. R. Starke: "Tuberculosis and Pregnancy," *Clinics in Chest Medicine 13*(4), pp. 693-707.

Vestal, K., and C. A. Mckenzie (Eds.): *High Risk Perinatal Nursing*, C. V. Mosby, Philadelphia, 1983.

Waterhouse, Lorraine: *Child Abuse and Child Abusers: Protection and Prevention*, Jessica Kingsley Publishers, Philadelphia, 1993.

Weiner, Susan: *Clinical Manual of Maternity and Gynecologic Nursing*, C. V. Mosby, Baltimore, 1989.

Whaley, Lucille F., and Donna L. Wong: *Essentials of Pediatric Nursing*, 4th ed., C. V. Mosby, St. Louis, 1993.

_______: *Nursing Care of Infants and Children*, 4th ed., Mosby Year Book, St. Louis, 1991.

Wong, Donna L., and Lucille F. Whaley: *Clinical Manual of Pediatric Nursing*, 3d ed., C. V. Mosby, St. Louis, 1990.

INDEX

INDEX

INDEX